£58-

Clinical Perspectives on Headache and Low Back Pain

Clinical Perspectives on Headache and Low Back Pain

Edited by

Claus Bischoff, Harald C. Traue, Helmuth Zenz
University of Ulm

Hogrefe & Huber Publishers
Toronto · Lewiston, NY · Göttingen · Bern

Library of Congress Cataloging-in-Publication Data

Clinical perspectives on headache and low back pain

Includes bibliographies and index.

1. Headache. 2. Backache. I. Bischoff, Claus, 1950– . II. Traue, Harald C., 1950– . III. Zenz, Helmut, 1939– .
[DNLM: 1. Backache. 2. Headache. WL 342 C641]
RB128.C57   1989   616.07'2   88-24424

Canadian Cataloguing in Publication Data

Clinical perspectives on headache and low back pain

Bibliography: p.
Includes index.

1. Headache. 2. Backache. I. Bischoff, Claus, 1950– . II. Traue, Harald C., 1950– . III. Zenz, Helmut, 1939– .
RC392.C58   1989   616.8'49   C88-094783-7

Copyright © 1989 by C. J. Hogrefe, Inc.

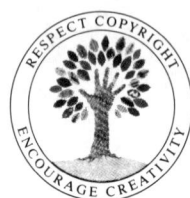

P.O. Box 51
Lewiston, NY 14092

12—14 Bruce Park Ave.
Toronto, Ontario M4P 2S3

No part of this book may be reproduced, stored in a retrieval system, or transmitted, in any form or by any means, electronic, mechanical, photocopying, microfilming, recording or otherwise, without written permission from the publisher.

Printed in Germany

ISBN 0-88937-025-7 Hogrefe · Toronto · Lewiston, NY · Göttingen · Zürich

ISBN 3-8017-0323-1 Hogrefe · Göttingen · Zürich · Toronto · Lewiston, NY

Editors' Foreword

Clinical Perspectives on Headache and Low Back Pain contains papers originally presented at a conference held at the University of Ulm on October 16 and 17, 1987. This conference was the continuation of a symposium that had taken place in Ulm five years previously (October 13—15, 1982), and that had dealt primarily with fundamental issues in headache research. The proceedings of that conference were subsequently published in 1983 by C. J. Hogrefe Publishers (Toronto/Lewiston, NY) under the title *Perspectives in Research on Headache*, edited by K.A. Holroyd, B.M. Schlote, and H. Zenz.

Both conferences were organized by the Department of Medical Psychology at the University of Ulm. Members of this department are involved in the project entitled "Psychophysiological Studies of Muscle Tension and Muscle Pain," part of the SFB 129 (Collaborative Research Program 129) funded by the German Research Foundation. This unit is an interdisciplinary group of researchers at the University of Ulm, who together have been taken a close look at psychotherapeutic processes using methods of social sciences, content analysis, and psychophysiology.

The aims of the Ulm Research Group in organizing the first conference were quite "selfish": Its members hoped to benefit extensively from the exchange with foreign scientists they invited and to be able to integrate much of this "foreign" knowledge into their own theoretical models and experimental approaches. Five years later we, as a research group, felt we were able to return part of what we had received. It was no small aim of the 1987 conference to present the principal results of our research to scientists of other universities in West Germany, Sweden, and the United States, and to seek out their detailed and constructive criticism. This explains why most of the papers in this volume have been contributed by researchers of the University of Ulm.

A further noticeable difference is already expressed in the title of the book: The general focus of psychophysiological pain research in West Germany—and in our research group, too—has shifted "downwards" from the head and neck toward the lower back and in some cases even toward the limbs. Approximately half of the contributions deal with low back pain. The concept of myogeny to explain pain is an important link between these research areas and thus occupies a relatively large place in this volume.

The Department of Medical Psychology and with it the University of Ulm gave much appreciated financial support to the conference; we were given additional financial support by the German Research Foundation, which also financed to a large extent the publication of this volume. The Board of the Collaborative Research Program 129 was particularly active in helping us to get the extra financial support: Our thanks to the chairperson of the Board, Professor Horst Kächele.

Once again, the C.J. Hogrefe Publishers, Göttingen and Toronto, has agreed to publish the proceedings of our conference. We should like to thank its representatives, especially Bernhard Otto and Dr. Michael Vogtmeier, with which we did the work involved in bringing out this book. We are grateful to Joseph A. Smith for his outstanding collaboration in editing the manuscripts.

Finally, we should like to thank the secretaries of the Department of Medical Psychology, Rita Lindenmayer, Hilde Böllert, Gaby Leibeling, and Martha Rissler, who typed most of the papers contributed by our department, and who did a remarkable job in organizing and typing everything concerned with the publication of this volume.

Ulm, West Germany, August 1988

Introduction

This volume contains papers originally presented at the Conference on Headache and Pain held in Ulm, West Germany, in 1987. Like an earlier volume of papers from a similar 1982 conference, this volume attempts to bridge a communication gap between European, particularly West German, researchers and their native English-speaking colleagues in America, Canada, Australia, and elsewhere. This communication gap may not be particularly salient to most American researchers; nonetheless, most of us can easily verify its existence simply by mentally reviewing our knowledge of current European pain research and clinical practice. European researchers, on the other hand, are acutely aware of this communication gap: While they have often made an admirable effort to remain current of the English-language literature, this effort is not widely reciprocated by American and other English-speaking researchers. Efforts to familiarize native English-speaking researchers with current European research are thus potentially quite valuable.

One unfortunate consequence of this communication gap is that differences in clinical practice and in the choice of research problems that should serve to stimulate further research advances may be ignored. The investigator who primarily reads the American and English literatures will find a number of provocative examples of differences between current concerns in these literatures and the emphasis of European researchers in this volume. One example is the research focus on the psychophysiology of pain, particularly the interest in the possible causal role of dysfunctional muscle activity in pain problems by West German researchers. This emphasis runs counter to recent trends in the American and English literatures, where studies on the psychophysiology of pain have been superceded by studies on pragmatic treatment issues in the psychological literature (see article by Andrasik). Moreover, recent concepts of pathophysiology (particularly in the medical literature) have tended to emphasize central variables, rather than peripheral variables (see Raskin, 1988, for example).

One benefit of the focus on peripheral muscle activity by European investigators is that it has stimulated these investigators to employ in pain research the technology for assessing electromyographic activity in the natural environment (e.g., the articles by Schlote and Bischoff/Müller). This technology remedies inherent limits of laboratory studies and has the potential to advance our understanding of the relationship between dysfunctional muscle activity and pain. Investigators in North America, England, and elsewhere with an interest in the psychophysiology of pain could benefit by embracing this methodological advance. On the other hand, European researchers might benefit from attention to the sort of pragmatic treatment issues that have occupied American researchers in recent years. Such pragmatic issues might involve the development of an assessment method for identifying myogenic pain sufferers and the demonstration that the diagnosis of myogenic pain has implications for treatment. Investigators in English-speaking countries, their European colleagues, and, ultimately, the chronic pain sufferer can only benefit from such mutual influence.

While about half this volume is devoted to research related to myogenic pain, a variety of other topics in the psychology of pain are addressed as well. Thus, readers in English-speaking countries can obtain at least a glimpse into current European research on psychological factors in pain. Hopefully this conference and the publication of the resulting papers will stimulate further exchange between researchers working in Europe and in English-speaking countries.

Kenneth A. Holyrod
Athens, Ohio, USA, July 1988

Reference

Raskin, N.H. (1988). On the origin of headpain. *Headache, 28*, 254—257.

Table of Contents

Preface v

Kenneth A. Holroyd
Introduction vii

SECTION A:
MYOGENIC FACTORS OF PAIN ETIOLOGY

Jeffrey Cram
Patterns of Neuromuscular Activity in Pain-Related Disorders 3

Claus Bischoff and Gerd Sauermann
Perception of Muscle Tension and Myogenic Headache:
A Signal-Detection Analysis 13

Harald C. Traue
Behavioral Inhibition in Stress Disorders and Myogenic Pain 29

Barbara Schlote
Long-Term Registration of Muscle Tension among Office Workers
Suffering from Tension Headache 46

Roland Teufel and Harald C. Traue
Myogenic Factors in Low Back Pain 64

SECTION B: DIAGNOSTIC PROCEDURES

Gabriele Manok and Helmuth Zenz
A Headache Interview 87

Gabriela Mendl and Christoph Stein
The German Version of the McGill Pain Questionnaire: The Münchner
Schmerzwortskala 123

SECTION C: PSYCHOSOCIAL FACTORS IN PAIN PERCEPTION AND PAIN MANAGEMENT

Monika Hasenbring
Psychological Predictors of Therapy Outcome in Chronic Low Back
Pain Patients 135

Peter Marschall, Ingrid Bowdler and Friedbert Rieth
Psychological Profiles of Chronic Pain Patients
and Factors Predisposing to the Development
of Pain-Induced Psychological Disorders 147

Roland Straub, Christfried Mayer and Walter Fröscher
Motivational and Volitional Characteristics of Patients with a
Prolapsed Intravertebral Disk and of Depressed Patients 166

SECTION D: PAIN MANAGEMENT

Frank Andrasik
Biofeedback Applications for Headache 181

Claus Bischoff and Klaus-Jürgen Müller
Portable EMG Biofeedback: A Single-Case Study
with a Muscle Contraction Headache Sufferer 201

Indexes 219

List of contributors

ANDRASIK, Frank, University of West Florida, Department of Psychology, College of Arts & Sciences, 11000 University Parkway, Pensacola, Florida 32514-5751, USA

BISCHOFF, Claus, Psychosomatische Fachklinik, Kurbrunnenstr. 12, 6702 Bad Dürkheim, FRG

BOWDLER, Ingrid, Schmerzambulanz der Abteilung für Anästhesiologie der Universität Ulm, Prittwitzstraße 43, 7900 Ulm, FRG

CRAM, Jeffrey R., Biofeedback Institute of Seattle, 901 Boren, Suite 1020, Seattle, Washington 98104, USA

FRÖSCHER, W., Psychiatrisches Landeskrankenhaus Weissenau, 7980 Ravensburg-Weissenau, FRG

HASENBRING, Monika, Klinikum der Christian-Albrechts-Universität Kiel, Abteilung Medizinische Psychologie, Zentrum Nervenheilkunde, Niemannsweg 147, 2300 Kiel 1, FRG

MAIER, Christfried, Psychiatrisches Landeskrankenhaus Weissenau, 7980 Ravensburg-Weissenau, FRG

MANOK, Gabi, Abteilung Medizinische Psychologie, Universität Ulm, Am Hochsträß 8, 7900 Ulm, FRG

MARSCHALL, Peter, Abteilung Medizinische Psychologie, Universität Ulm, Am Hochsträß 8, 7900 Ulm, FRG

MENDL, Gabriela, Klinkum Großhadern, Abteilung für Anästhesiologie, 8000 München, FRG

MÜLLER, Klaus-Jürgen, Institut für Sport und Sportwissenschaft, Universität Freiburg, Schwarzwaldstr. 175, 7800 Freiburg, FRG

RIETH, Friedbert, Riedhauserstr. 59, 7983 Wilhelmsdorf, FRG

SAUERMANN, Gerd, Otto-Wagner-Str. 14, 8034 Germaring, FRG

SCHLOTE, Barbara, Klinikum Mannheim, Theodor-Kurtzer-Ufer, 6800 Mannheim, FRG

STEIN, Christoph, Klinikum Großhadern, Abteilung für Anästhesiologie, 8000 München, FRG

STRAUB, Roland, Psychiatrisches Landeskrankenhaus Weissenau, 7980 Ravensburg-Weissenau, FRG

TEUFEL, Roland, Forschungsstelle für Psychotherapie, Christian-Belser-Str. 79a, 7000 Stuttgart 70, FRG

TRAUE, Harald C., Forschungsstelle für Psychotherapie, Christian-Belser-Str. 79a, 7000 Stuttgart 70, FRG

ZENZ, Helmuth, Abteilung Medizinische Psychologie, Universität Ulm, Am Hochsträß 8, 7900 Ulm, FRG

SECTION A:
MYOGENIC FACTORS OF PAIN ETIOLOGY

Patterns of Neuromuscular Activity in Pain-Related Disorders

Jeffrey R. Cram

This study favors a myogenic model of back pain. Its basic assumption is that in describing back pain processes, one must also assess patterns of neuromuscular activity and not only the activity of single muscle sites. This seems to be true because pain possibly migrates as a result of protective guarding, and because pain may be referred from damaged muscle tissue to unaffected sites. The study develops and examines the role of muscle site, posture, and symmetry in describing patterns of neuromuscular activity in pain-related disorders. Two hundred patients with chronic back, shoulder, or neck pain were examined in a sitting and standing position regarding the muscle activity of eleven sites of the back, neck, and head region. The EMG of these muscle sites was registered on the left side and on the right side with an electromyograph simply placed over the muscle in question without affixing the electrodes.

The level of neuromuscular activity turns out to be greater while standing than while sitting; it is greater on the left than on the right side. A significant increase in the level of muscle activity while subjects are standing is noted for the trapezius and the L3 paraspinal muscle site. This is especially true for the left side. The higher muscle activity on the left may be due to the fact that most subjects are righthanded, which requires compensation for gravity (biomechanical model). Perhaps it is a manifestation of the dominance of the right hemisphere with respect to negative emotions (emotional model). Interestingly, the muscle group bearing most of the "effort" is the T10 paraspinal muscle group. The activity of this muscle group shows for either posture the most robust correlation with the total amount of muscle activity. A case study demonstrates that multiple scanning of neuromuscular activation patterns is both of statistical and of clinical significance.

The nature of the etiology of cervical and back pain is very complex. However, it is estimated that 80% of neck and back pain is attributed to postural or mechanical causes, rather than discogenic or other medical etiologies (Kraus & Raab, 1961; Hollinghead, 1976; Calliet, 1979). Since the primary function of the muscles of the back and neck is postural support, a better understanding and assessment of the pattern of organization of these muscles would contribute to our understanding of the myogenic contributions to back pain.

When a human stands in an erect fashion, the body is subjected to gravitational influences according to the laws of Newtonian physics. If the body is aligned over its center of gravity, the weight of the body is borne primarily on the bones and ligaments, and very little muscular effort is needed (Carmichael & Burkart, 1979). The major force of muscular support during standing is found in the soleus muscle groups (Calliet, 1977). However, as lifestyle demands, work, and emotional display patterns emerge, throwing one off of one's center of gravity, the muscles of the back must come into play to keep him erect. Over a prolonged period of time, this may place habitual patterns of strain on the bones, ligaments, and muscles, creating the internal environment from which neck and back pain may emerge. The sensory origin of this pain may be found in the bones, the nerves, the vessels, or the muscles and soft tissue (Calliet, 1977).

The origins of myogenic neck and back pain may initially be attributed to other disorders. For example, a mechanical source of pain may mandate that the muscles in the afflicted region clamp down in a "splinting" fashion to immobilize the area and prevent further damage (Price, 1948). This sustained tonic contraction leads to diminished blood flow (ischemia) and the buildup of lactic acid, both of which stimulate the nociceptor in the muscle itself (Rodbard, 1975). This initial splinting may persist beyond the initial acute phase of the injury due to the development of a pain-spasm-pain cycle (Bonica, 1957). Lastly, the patient may develop a habitual neuromuscular pattern of "protective guarding": The patient learns to favor the site of pain, thus activating muscle groups that move the body away from the pain itself. The neuromuscular dysfunction, and therefore pain, migrates to a site away from the pain itself (Price, 1948).

The origins of myogenic pain may also be lie in irritation of the muscle tissue itself (Kellgren, 1937). Strains, sprains, and other trauma of the muscle tissue may result in necrosis of fibers within a muscle, leading to the development of a palpable painful nodules (Kraus & Raab, 1961; Sola & Williams, 1956). The perception of this pain may be "referred" to a muscle site some distance from the "trigger point" or nodule (Travell & Rinzler, 1952).

The assessment protocols for describing the patterns of organization for painful neck and back muscles are poorly developed. In physical therapy, a gross assessment for strength and range of motion may be done, but, unfortunately, these may be difficult to quantify and may lack sensitivity. Wolf, Basmajian, Russe, and Kutner (1979), for example, note that a limited range of motion in otherwise healthy individuals may be attributed to their sedate lifestyle.

Surface electromyographic assessment techniques have also been conducted in a time-series fashion to assess the erector spinea muscles during quiet standing and dynamic movement (Wolf & Basmajian, 1978). While this technique may adequately describe neuromuscular dysfunctions for a single muscle group, it provides very little information concerning the status of other adjacent or even distant muscle groups. Sampling from multiple muscle groups may be of clinical importance. Price (1948), for example, has observed that neuromuscular activation patterns may migrate away from the actual site of pain. Such migration patterns would be missed using a single site of study. In addition, it is well known that the back muscles are well orchestrated (Hollinghead, 1976). Thus, alterations in muscular activity and posture in the low back would certainly result in compensatory changes in the muscles of the upper back and neck.

This article develops and examines the role of muscle site, posture, and symmetry in describing patterns of neuromuscular activity and pain-related disorders. It presents an assessment procedure that systematically samples from the right and left aspects of eleven muscle sites, in the two static postures of unsup-

Variable	Levels	Clinical concept
Muscle site	11	Sites of activation
Symmetry	2	Splinting or guarding
Posture	2	Postural disturbance

Table 1. Clinical concepts investigated.

ported sitting and quiet standing (see Table 1). By examining this type of data base, patterns of neuromuscular activity may more accurately identify the muscle group(s) involved; asymmetrical patterns may suggest splinting or guarding; and the postural variables may clarify the impact of posture in pain-related disorder.

Method

Subjects

The sample consisted of 200 consecutive admissions of chronic pain patients to the Swedish Hospital Medical Center inpatient pain Therapy Program. The primary symptom of 69% of the sample was that of low back pain; 12% presented with shoulder pain, 9% with neck pain, and 10% had pain in other areas. Their mean age was 42.5 years; 51% were male and 49% female.

Instrumentation

Surface electromyographic activity from the muscular system was recorded using a J & J electromyograph (Model M-53). The instrument had an input impedance of 100 MΩ and a bandpass filtering network of 100 to 200 Hz. The raw EMG audio function was selected to allow for detection of electrical noise and biological artifact. The preamplifier of the system was located externally, at the electrode site. Two silver chloride (posts) style electrodes, 10 mm in diameter, separated by 2 cm, were plugged directly into the preamplifier. These served as the active electrodes. The reference ground was attached to the bony prominence of the wrist and connected to the preamplifier by a 36-inch lead. EMG activity was quantified using a digital integrator (J & J, Model D-200). This instrument integrated the muscle activity over a 2-second period of time, presenting the information every 2 seconds in a serial updating fashion.

Procedure

EMG activity was collected using the sampling procedure previously described by Cram and Steger (1983), and Cram (1986). In essence, the procedure was as follows: The post-style active electrodes were lightly coated with Beckman Electrode Paste and placed over the muscle site of interest, making direct contact with the skin. They were not affixed, but held motionless over the site by hand with a light pressure. No skin preparation was done except in the case of obvious need (e.g., excessively dry or oily skin or make-up). The electrodes were left on the site for some 6 to 12 seconds, or until the EMG activity had stabilized. The EMG activity was considered stable when each successive data point was within 10% of each other. The best two samples were recorded and utilized in further analysis.

The right and left aspect of eleven muscle sites were samples, first in the sitting and then in the standing posture. The location and electrode placement of the sites may be seen in Figures 1 and 2. The abdominal site (not shown in the figures), was located 3 cm to the right and left of the umbilicus. With the exception of the frontalis site, the electrode configuration ran parallel to the muscle fibers of the muscles of interest. A total of 44 samples of muscle activity (11 sites × 2 sides × 2 postures) were collected on each patient. The sequence of the scanning procedure was as follows: The muscles of the face and anterior aspect of the neck (SCM) were sampled first in the sitting posture. The patients were simply asked to sit sideways on a flat-bottomed office chair with their hands in the lap, with no support given to the back. The patients were asked to sit comfortably. They were then asked to stand comfortably with the hands at the side, while the same sites were sampled again using the electrode paste residue left behind from the first scan to assist in the replication of placement. The patients

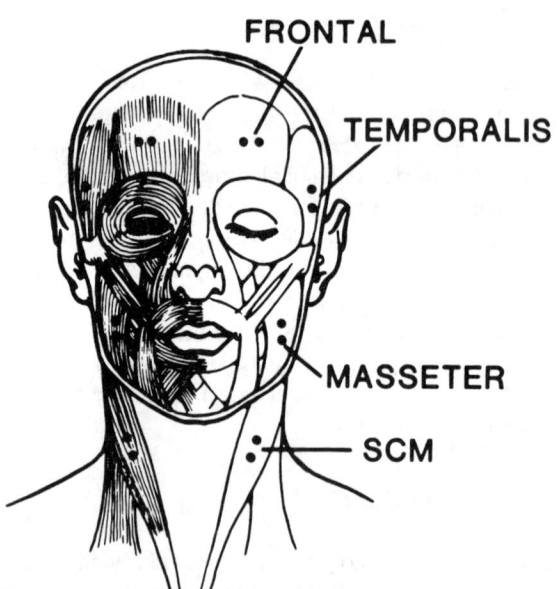

Figure 1. Scan sites for the face. (From Cram and Engstrom, 1986; reproduced by permission.)

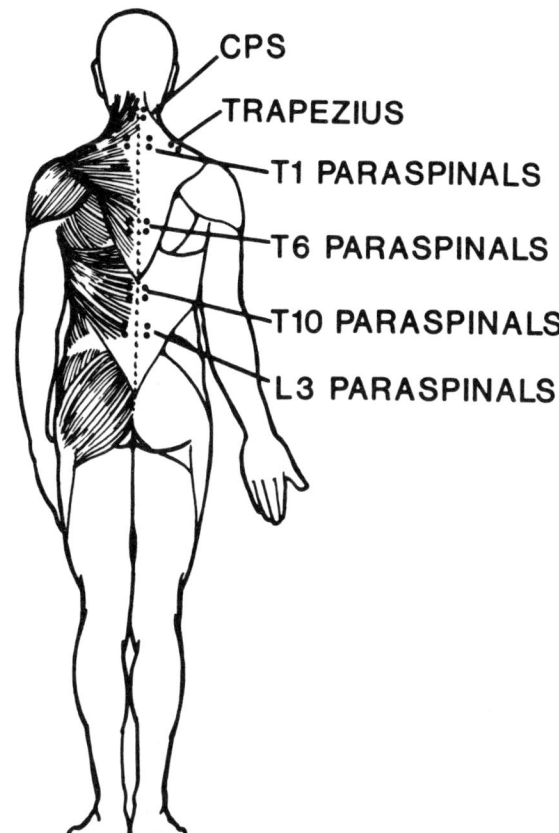

Figure 2. Scan sites for the back. (From Cram and Engstrom, 1986; reproduced by permission.)

were then asked to sit again in the same fashion, and the muscles of the posterior aspect of the neck and the back and abdomen were sampled. They were then asked to stand while these sites were sampled a second time. The total time for this procedure was approximately 15 to 20 minutes.

Results

The 44 samples of EMG activity were submitted to an analysis of variance (ANOVA) with repeated measures. The within variables were as follows: Muscle Site (11); Symmetry (2); and Posture (2). All posteriori tests were conducted using Tukeys (HSD) at the .05 level.

The means and standard deviations of the EMG activity of each muscle site for the entire sample are presented in Table 2. The analysis of variance indicated a significant effect for Muscle Site (F = 44.3, p < .000); Posture (F = 32.6,

Table 2. Means and standard deviations of each muscle site.

Muscle site		Sit Left	Sit Right	Stand Left	Stand Right
Frontalis	x̄	2.58	2.54	2.39	2.38
	SD	2.42	2.41	1.67	1.58
Temporalis		3.82	3.65	3.39	3.28
		4.52	3.70	3.98	3.42
Masseter		2.16	1.96	1.80	1.73
		2.51	1.81	1.59	1.87
SCM		1.49	1.33	1.34	1.35
		1.69	1.34	1.11	1.44
CPS		2.79	2.59	2.28	2.12
		1.52	1.51	1.78	1.12
Trapezius		2.71	3.10	5.31	4.63
		3.84	5.03	5.53	5.45
Paraspinal T_1		2.69	2.77	3.53	3.27
		1.66	1.78	3.51	3.18
Paraspinal T_6		3.86	3.43	2.96	3.10
		3.72	3.65	3.88	4.01
Paraspinal T_{10}		3.30	2.58	3.90	3.32
		3.25	2.71	4.19	3.66
Paraspinal L_3		2.38	2.17	4.70	4.60
		4.32	3.03	5.44	4.19
Abdominal		1.19	1.21	1.33	1.33
		1.83	1.23	1.07	1.09

$p < .000$); Symmetry ($F = 18.1$, $p < .000$); Muscle Site × Posture ($F = 35.3$, $p < .000$); and Muscle Site × Posture × Symmetry ($F = 3.5$, $p < .00$).

A finer analysis of this data indicates that the level of neuromuscular activity was significantly greater while standing compared to sitting. The left aspect of the neuromuscular system was significantly greater than the right. Investigation of the interaction between muscle site and posture revealed a significant increase in the level of neuromuscular activity during the standing posture for the trapezius and the L3 paraspinal muscle sites. When the Muscle Site × Posture × Symmetry interaction was investigated, the left aspect of trapezius and the L3 paraspinal muscle groups were observed to be significantly more elevated during standing compared to the right aspect. A left-sided dominance is noted in the T10 paraspinal muscles in both the sitting and standing postures. The T6 paraspinal muscles were significantly more elevated on the left aspect as well, but only in the sitting posture.

Discussion

The back and neck pain patients in this study clearly demonstrate that patterns of neuromuscular activity varied consistently from one posture to another, from one muscle site to another, and in an asymmetrical fashion. Symmetry appeared to be a very significant issue, with the left aspect of the back playing a substantial role in terms of activation patterns. Posture appeared to effect muscle groups in a differential fashion. Interestingly enough, the T6 paraspinals tended to show a greater amount of left-sided activation while sitting compared to standing. The trapezius and L3 paraspinal muscles, on the other hand, tended to show a greater level of left-sided activation while standing compared to sitting. The T10 paraspinals indicated left-sided activation patterns for both sitting and standing. Left-sided dominance observed at all of the active sites.

In most surface EMG studies of pain, the site of recording is held constant. The investigator hereby assumes that the selected site adequately represents the myogenic contribution to pain being assessed. This assumption is typically hidden, seldom mentioned in the discussion of the findings, and yet contributes greatly to the data base and the understanding of myogenic pain. Goldstein (1972), after reviewing the psychophysiological literature on surface EMG, emphasized the importance of "sampling" from the neuromuscular system. In addition, the concept of "referred pain" (Travell & Rinzler, 1952) mandates that the investigation of pain go beyond the reported site of pain. Lastly, Price, Clare and Ewerhardt (1948) observed the migration of muscle activation patterns in back pain patients. Such a migration may be reflective of an individual patient moving from a "muscle splinting" pattern, to one better understood as a "protective guarding" pattern in which the person uses the muscles to move away from pain, favoring the injured site. All of these issues point to the importance of muscle site as a variable.

If one were to "assume" that one muscle group bears most of the "effort," it would be the T10 paraspinal muscle group. In the present study, this group received no postural relief with activation patterns occurring in both postures. In a related study (Cahn & Cram, 1987), both individual muscle groups and "regions" were correlated to the total amount of EMG activity summed from all EMG scan sites in a primarily back pain population. Some of the finding from this study are presented in Table 3. As can be seen, the upper and lower back carry most of the weight. The T10 site, however, shows the most robust correlation for both postures. These findings were found to be independent of statistical artifact or redundancy; they suggest that stronger clinical information might be found at the T10, rather than the L3 muscle sites. Further consideration needs to be given as to which muscle sites are "traditionally" monitored. In addition, specific attention might be directed at the T10 paraspinal group. The structural and functional aspects of these finding needs to be described.

The role of symmetry would appear to be of clinical importance as well. The left-sided dominance of activation patterns in the back muscles of the pain popu-

Region	Sit	Stand
Face	.54	.38
Neck	.63	.42
Upper back	.72	.76
Lower back	.79	.76
Abdominal	.57	.35
Muscle groups		
Cervical	.50	.40
Trapezius	.49	.50
T1 Paraspinals	.63	.59
T6 Paraspinals	.54	.59
T10 Paraspinals	.72	.73
L3 Paraspinals	.65	.54

Table 3. Correlations between regions or muscle groups and total muscle activity (adapted from Cahn & Cram, 1987).

lation was clearly evidenced in this study and related studies (Cram & Engstrom, 1986). The role of the left side of the back as the most sensitive indicator of neuromuscular dysfunction needs to be explored. The most parsimonious model would be that of a biomechanical model. Here, one would assume that the population as a whole is right-handed. As they reach out to operate their world from this right-handed perspective, the left aspect of the back would then come into play as they move off their center of gravity. Over the natural history of use of the back, the left aspect would therefore be more available to both over use patterns as well as injury. A second model would be an "emotional" model. Ferenczi (1926), for example, observed that hysteria tends to present itself most commonly on the left aspect of the body. Davidson and Fox (1982) have documented that the right hemisphere of the brain tends to be the one that handles negatively valenced emotions. It is possible that pain or pain-related emotions are represented in the right hemisphere, and therefore the left aspect of the body. Flor, Turk, and Birbaumer (1985) have proposed an interactive diathesis stress model in which the "weakened" muscular structures become the common avenues for stress-related responses. Further research on both the biomechanical as well as the emotional aspects may clarify this left-sided finding in the future.

The role of posture in the assessment of pain-related disorders cannot be overlooked. In the current study, posture was found to effect muscle groups in a differential fashion. The T6 paraspinals were more activated during sitting, the trapezius and L3 paraspinals were more activated during standing, and the T10 were activated in both postures. While this study is focused primarily on the "static" nature of the neuromuscular system, posture should also be considered from the "dynamic" aspect as well. Wolf and Basmajian (1978) clearly demonstrated abnormal recruitment patterns in back pain patients as they go into forward flexion or during rotational patterns with the pelvis stabilized. The clinician/researcher should be aware of a revived interest in biomechanical or postural models of back pain (Dolce & Raczynski, 1985).

The clinical utility of an EMG muscle-scanning procedure for the assessment of muscle site, symmetry, and posture is perhaps most clearly seen in individual case study. Table 4 presents a protocol on a 36-year-old caucasian male who has a primary pain complaint of low back pain of six-month duration. The findings of the study are not subtle: As one reviews the columns of data, one clearly sees activation patterns at the T10 and L3 sites; asymmetrical patterns, indicating a left-sided dominance, are also clearly present. Lastly, one can easily see that when the patient bears weight upon standing, this merely accentuates the site

Table 4. Data from muscle scanning protocol on a 36-year-old low back pain patient.

Muscle site	Sit		Stand	
	Left	Right	Left	Right
Frontalis	3.3	3.5*	2.1	2.3
Temporalis	2.4	2.6	1.9	2.1
Masseter	0.6	0.7	0.5	0.7
SCM	0.5	0.5	0.6	0.6
Cervical	1.5	2.0	2.0	2.1
Trapezius	2.2	2.2	3.1	3.0
T1 Paraspinal	1.7	2.0	1.8	11.9
T6 Paraspinal	3.7	3.3	4.0	4.1
T10 Paraspinal	19.7*	9.2*	62.7*	43.9*
L3 Paraspinal	8.6	2.6	28.8*	18.5*
Abdominal	0.5	0.7	0.4	0.6

and symmetry findings. Perhaps one of the more interesting aspects of this individual patient's findings is that his low back pain is described as being perceived in the L3 to L5 region. However, the highest level of activation is seen somewhat higher in the T10 region of the back. Perhaps this documents what Price (1948) described as migration of activation patterns to sites away from pain.

The data presented support both the statistical and clinical significance of studied concepts. In the last few years, there has been an increasing interest in "patterns" of muscle activity (Dolce & Raczynski, 1985; Noewen & Bush, 1983). While this paper presents the "static" aspects of these patterns, dynamic elements should also be considered.

References

Bonica, J.J. (1957). Introduction to symposium on pain. *Archives of Surgery, 112,* 732—738.
Cahn T.S., & Cram, J.R. (1987). *Relationship between muscle regions and average total muscle activity: Support for the back.* Presented at the convention of the Biofeedback Society of America, Boston.
Calliet, R. (1977). *Soft tissue injury and disability.* Philadelphia: Davis.

Calliet, R. (1979). *The low back syndrome*. Philadelphia: Davis.
Carmichael, S. W., & Burkart, S.L. (1979). Clinical anatomy of the lumbar complex. *Physical Therapy, 59*, 966—968.
Cram, J.R., & Steger, J.C. (1983). EMG Scanning in the diagnosis of chronic pain. *Biofeedback and Self-Regulation, 8*, 229—241.
Cram, J.R., & Engstrom, D. (1986). Patterns of neuromuscular activity pain and non-pain patients. *Clinical Biofeedback and Health, 9*, 106—115.
Cram, J.R. (1986). *Clinical EMG: Muscle scanning and diagnostic manual for surface recordings*. Seattle: Clinical Resources.
Davidson, R.J., & Fox, N.A. (1982). Asymmetrical brain activity discriminates between positive and negative stimuli in human infants. *Science, 218*, 1235—1237.
Dolce, J.J., & Raczynski, J.M. (1985). Neuromuscular activity and electromyography in painful backs: Psychological and biomechanical model in assessment and treatment. *Psychological Bulletin, 97*, 502—520.
Ferenczi, S. (1926). An attempted explanation of some hysterical stigmata. In S. Ferenczi (Ed.), *Further contribution to the theory and technique of psychoanalysis* (pp. 110—117). London: Hogarth.
Flor, H., Turk, D.C., & Birbaumer, N. (1985). Assessment of stress-related psychophysiological reactions in chronic back pain patients. *Journal of Consulting and Clinical Psychology, 53*, 354—364.
Goldstein, B. (1972). Electromyography: A measure of skeletal muscle response. In N. Greenfield & Sternbach, R. (Eds.), *Handbook of psychophysiology*. New York: Holt, Reinhart, and Winston.
Hollinghead, W.H. (1976). *Functional anatomy of the limbs and back*. Philadelphia: Saunders.
Kellgren, J.H. (1937). Observations on referred pain arising from muscles. *Clinical Science, 3*, 175—190.
Kraus H., & Raab, W. (1961). *Hypokinetic disease*. Springfield, IL: Charles C. Thomas.
Noewen A., & Bush, C. (1983). The relationship between EMG and chronic low back pain. *Pain, 20*, 109—123.
Price, J.P., Clare, M.H., & Ewerhardt, R.H. (1948). Studies in low backache with persistent muscle spasm. *Archives of physical medicine and rehabilitation, 19*, 703—709.
Rodbard, S. (1975). Pain in contracting muscles. In B.L. Crue (Ed), *Pain: Research and treatment*. New York: Academic Press.
Sola A.E., & Williams, R.L. (1956). Myofacial pain syndromes. *Neurology, 6*, 91—95.
Travell, J., & Rinzler, S. (1952). The myofascial genesis of pain. *Postgraduate Medicine, 11*, 425—434.
Wolf S., & Basmajian, J.V. (1978). Assessment of paraspinal electromyographic activity in normal subjects and chronic back pain patients using a muscle biofeedback device. In E. Asmussen & K. Jorgensen (Eds.), *International Series on Biomechanics, Vol. 6b*. Baltimore: University Park Press.
Wolf, S., Basmajian, J.V., Russe, T.C., & Kutner, M. (1979). Normative data on low back mobility and activity levels. *American Journal of Physical Medicine, 58*, 217—229.

Perception of Muscle Tension and Myogenic Headache: A Signal-Detection Analysis

Claus Bischoff and Gerd Sauermann

We hypothesize that individuals suffering from myogenic headache have conditioned perceptual deficits concerning their muscle tension: (1) They are less able than normals to rate their muscle tension correctly because of a diminished perceptual capacity; (2) they have a bias toward ignoring actually occurring changes in muscle tension; and (3) they tend to give cautious responses as to whether the actual muscle tension is changing or not.

In order to test these assumptions, we conducted a signal-detection experiment. The proprioceptive stimuli were defined by means of optical feedback. Each subject was instructed to contract voluntarily the forehead muscle to such an extent that a green light went on; subjects were requested to note the amount of muscle contraction necessary to turn on the light and to compare it with a second contraction necessary to turn on the light again. Eighty trials of this type were conducted. In half of the trials the first and the second contraction had to be equally high, while in the other half a well-defined different muscle tension was necessary to turn on the second light. Subjects had to judge whether or not there was a difference between the two contractions of a trial. Trial presentation was controlled automatically. We used this experimental procedure to study 12 subjects suffering from myogenic headache, 15 migraineurs, and 12 pain-free controls.

Subjects suffering from myogenic headache proved to be less sensitive and more cautious than both migraineurs and pain-free controls. This confirms our hypotheses. Unexpectedly, both headache groups had a tendency to accentuate differences between muscle tension. Possible reasons of these results and the perceptual deficit in general are discussed.

Practitioners, orthopedics, and physiotherapists often maintain that individuals suffering from tension headache are not able to recognize when their muscles are tense. Similar hypotheses can be found in the headache literature. Birbaumer (1975) interprets tension headache as a consequence of lacking proprioception which is acquired and maintained by positive or negative reinforcement. Whereas Birbaumer adopts an operant conditioning model, Fowler and Kraft (1974) explain the perceptual deficit in terms of adaptation to a permanent stimulus. They compare the patient with chronic neck and shoulder pain with "a

---

The research was carried out with the support of the German Research Foundation (DFG) in the Special Research Unit 129 ("Psychotherapeutic Processes") at the University of Ulm, West Germany. The authors wish to thank B. Dahme, G. Fehm-Wolfsdorf, H.C. Traue, and Helmuth Zenz for critical and constructive comments on an earlier draft of this paper, and P. Zintl for the translation of the manuscript.

boiler factory worker who has worked around noise so long he does not hear it anymore. Our patients with chronic tension pain appeared not to 'hear' the background of high muscle activity" (p. 28). As an exception, Epstein and Cinciripini (1981) think it possible that individuals suffering from tension headache are *hyper*sensitive to small changes in muscle activity. In the acquisition phase, changes of muscle activity would usually preceed tension headaches. Hence, these changes may become discriminative stimuli for the report of pain when the report is positively or negatively reinforced. For this reason, the report of pain no longer needs a physiological basis.

Only a few empirical investigations consider the perception of muscle activity in individuals suffering from tension headache. The subjects of Fowler and Kraft (1974) estimated their neck muscle tension several times while reading a magazine and filling in a personality questionnaire. For judging they used an 11-point rating scale. The ratings were correlated intraindividually with the corresponding EMG values of the neck muscle activity. The mean correlation reached significance neither in the experimental group with subjects suffering from neck and shoulder pain nor in the pain-free control group. However, the mean values of the EMG and its variability during the experimental situation are far from being representative of the trapezius activity in everyday life (cf. Schlote, in this volume). Especially in the control group is the muscle activity very low ($\bar{x}= 3.1\,\mu V/s$) and varies only to a minimal extent ($s = 0.9\,\mu V/s$). Why, then, should these subjects perceive changes in muscle activity when muscle activity does not vary and they are not tensed at all?

Blanchard and collegues (Blanchard, Jurish, Andrasik, & Epstein, 1981; Appelbaum, Blanchard, & Andrasik, 1984) used the magnitude production method of Stevens (1975) with the specifications of Stilson, Matus, and Ball (1980) to operationalize the perceptual capacities of headache sufferers. The subject's muscle tension during instruction was designated as a modulus (Figure 6). By isometric contraction, each subject successively had to produce other tension levels corresponding to figures between 4 and 30. As a parameter of perceptual precision, the intraindividual correlation between the muscle activity produced (the EMG) and the muscle activity to be produced (the figures) was computed. The correlations were calculated on the basis of the psychophysiological function that fitted best the relationship between the two variables. The correlations proved to be highly significant. However, the two experiments yielded to conflicting results. In the study of 1981, the activity of the forearm muscles—the only muscles being considered—was discriminated best by the subjects of the control group ($\bar{r} = 0.76$), followed by the subjects of a tension headache group ($\bar{r} = 0.68$), subjects suffering from combined migraine and tension headache ($r = 0.60$), and finally the migraineurs ($\bar{r} = 0.51$). The second experiment did not replicate this difference, though a significant difference regarding frontal and neck muscle activity was found. In this study, the migraineurs proved to be most precise ($\bar{r} = 0.88$), followed by subjects with combined headache ($\bar{r} = 0.84$), and tension headache sufferers ($\bar{r} = 0.71$). Control group data do not exist.

The method of direct scaling as applied in Blanchard's experiments has two shortcomings. First, the modulus was not standardized to a defined muscle activity between individual minimum and maximum, so that systematic differences between the range of activity levels to be discriminated could account for the results (the higher the tension level the worse the perceptual capacity; cf. Stilson, Matus, & Ball, 1980; Bischoff, 1989). Moreover, the direct scaling method does not allow for differentiating the individual's precision on different tension levels, which may be quite variable (Bischoff, 1989).

The synopsis shows that perception of muscle tension is investigated with very different methods and under various experimental conditions. Therefore, the differing results are not astonishing. In assessing perceptual precision, it is important to consider not only the tension level and the tension range the data are relating to,x but also the muscles included as well as the quality and extent of additional external stimulation. It is of special significance whether the contractions investigated are voluntarily produced or spontaneously fluctuating. The results may depend on the signal characteristics—levels vs. differentials—the experimenter explores. Moreover, results may be influenced by biases. The experiments presented above do not distinguish biases from true sensory capacities.

There is still another problem with the described studies which deserves attention: the diagnostic procedures applied. "Tension headache" is implicitly thought to be a "myogenic headache"—a headache caused by dysfunctionally high muscle activity. For myogenic headache sufferers it would be important to have correct perception of muscle activity in order to avoid or to stop in time irregularly high muscle tension which, when continued, would produce headache. But Fowler and Kraft (1974) as well as Blanchard and colleagues do not assure the myogeny of their subjects' headache. They use the common procedure of diagnosing tension headache: by excluding vascular and organic headaches. As shown in an earlier paper (Bischoff & Traue, 1983), only a subgroup of these "tension headache" sufferers suffer from true myogenic headache.

The subject matter of our experiment on tension perception is as follows: Though we do not have a really satisfying solution for the diagnostic problem either (see below), our study refers to myogenic headache. The muscle activities under consideration are relatively short voluntary contractions of the frontal muscle. The tension levels remain under 20% of the individual tension maximum. This range of muscle tension is observed in individuals suffering from myogenic headache and pain-free controls in everyday situations (cf. Schlote, in this volume; Sauermann, 1986).

Several experimental studies favor the trapezius muscle as being more relevant in myogenic headache than the frontal muscle (Traue, Mahoney, & Bischoff, 1985b). We decided to use the frontal muscle for practical reasons. Because of the many degrees of freedom of the joints involved, defined contractions of the trapezius muscle cannot reliably be reproduced. Therefore, equal EMG values may have different meanings.

In order to discriminate between sensory capacity and biases, we developed a signal-detection design, which allows for testing three aspects of the perceptual deficit hypothesis:

Individuals suffering from myogenic headache

1) are less able than individuals not suffering from this symptom to rate their muscle tension correctly because of a diminished perceptual capacity;
2) they have a bias toward ignoring actually occurring changes in muscle tension;
3) they have a bias toward uncertainty, that is, they tend to give cautious responses whether the actual muscle tension is changing or not.

Method

Subjects

Thirty-nine subjects participated in the experiment, 12 of which were suffering from myogenic headache, 15 were migraineurs, and 12 were pain-free controls. The three groups were comparable with respect to age and sex. All subjects were undergraduate medical students. They received DM 30 for their participation. A total of 200 students of medical psychology at the University of Ulm, FRG, completed a *Headache Information Survey*. In case of doubt, the diagnosis according to this survey was revised on the basis of a clinical interview. The control group consisted of subjects reporting that they never or only infrequently had headache or sensations of tightness and pressure in the head and neck area. The subjects of the headache groups reported suffering from headache at least several times per month. The mean headache intensity was at least four on a visual analogue scale which was subsequently subdivided into ten intervals. All subjects were tested in a headache-free state.

At present, a *positive* diagnosis of myogenic headache, i.e., the proof of the myogeny of a headache, is theoretically possible but quite difficult to realize (Bischoff & Traue, 1983; Bischoff & Müller, in this volume; Pikoff, 1984). For this reason, myogenic headache was diagnosed by a forced exclusion procedure. Headaches with the following symptoms: throbbing quality, sudden onset, prodromal, and other typically vascular symptoms, were classified as migraine. All individuals in the myogenic headache group reported feelings of pain in the neck, the frontal or temporal region. The headaches were of tense and dull quality, slowly developing and fading away. In no case did a subject of this group exhibit vascular symptoms. In contrast, subjects of the migraine headache group possibly suffered from muscular symptoms as well. Vegetative symptoms (nausea, vomiting, etc.) did not count as indicative of migraine because they may be a consequence of strong pain of any origin. The same is true for unilaterality, which also may occur in myogenic headache (Wolf-Cramer, 1984). No subject suffered from constant headache of the depressive type; no subject took analgesics. The headaches did not seem to be under operant control (Fordyce, 1976). The experiment was conducted under double-blind conditions. The two experimenters tested about the same number of subject in each experimental group.

Procedure

Subjects were contacted individually. Initially, the experimenter gave a short explanation of the experiment, and fixed the leads at the frontal muscle. In the first phase, the minimum activity of the frontal muscle was assessed. The minimum activity was registered with the eyes open following some selected exercises of Jacobson's (1983) progressive muscle relaxation training. The minimum was the basis for the definition of the stimuli in the signal detection experiment, the second experimental phase. This phase consisted of 84 trials, 4 training trials, and 80 valid trials, which were administered in blocks of 20 trials. Between the blocks the subject had some time to recover. Each trial consisted of two defined contractions and a following judgement comparing the two contractions with respect to their equal or different intensity.

Structure of a Trial

A major problem in signal-detection experiments on interoceptive stimuli is the definition of signal and noise. We defined signal and noise by means of optical feedback. The subject obtained the stimuli by producing them. The task (cf. Figures 1 and 2) was to raise the eyebrows voluntarily, thereby contracting the frontal muscle.

Subjects had to raise the eyebrows to such an extent that a green light went on. They were instructed to keep the muscle tension in the "green interval" as long as possible and to sense the amount of muscle tension necessary to produce the green light. They were informed by a red light when they exceeded the required tension, and by a yellow light when the tension was too low. The subjects had to produce "green" for two seconds altogether—the computer added up the times the subjects remained in the interval. At the end of the two seconds the subjects no longer got optical feedback; rather, they were instructed to relax the muscle to a critical relaxation level. Once they had reached this level, they had to contract the muscle again to such an extent as to produce "green" once more. The two contractions of a trial producing green were either equally high or differed to a well-defined extent. In terms of signal detection theory, trials with two equally high contractions are noise-alone trials (see Figure 1), and trials with two different contractions are signal-plus-noise trials (see Figure 2).

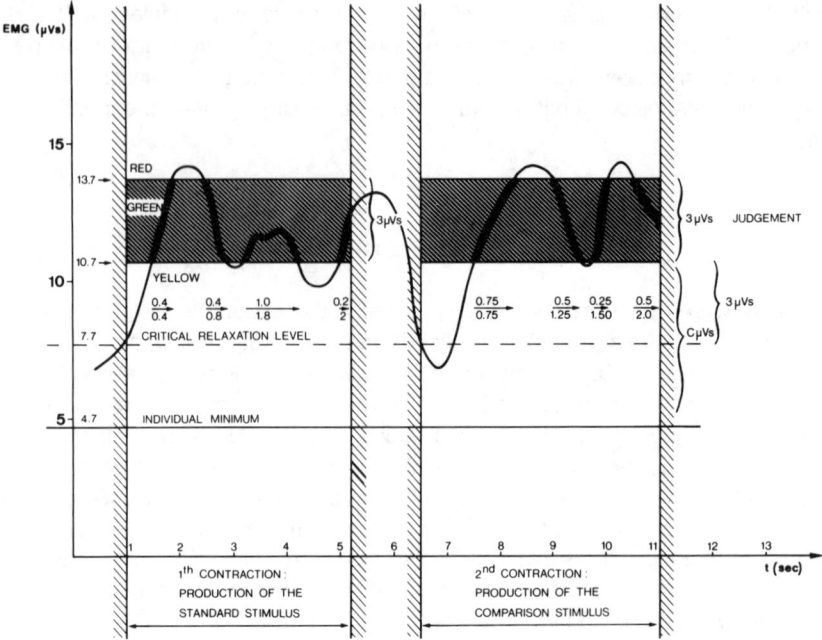

Figure 1. One possible trial of the signal detection experiment: Noise alone.

Noise-alone trials and signal-plus-noise trials followed each other randomly. In signal-plus-noise trials, either the first contraction producing green (standard stimulus) was smaller than the second one (comparison stimulus; this case is shown in Figure 2), or vice versa (not shown) in random sequence. The green intervals represented a contraction range of three µV/s. In signal-plus-noise trials, the difference between the two contractions producing green was 4.5 µV/s. In noise-alone trials, the lower limit of the required contractions was always 6 µV/s higher than the individual minimum assessed in the first experimental phase. In signal-plus-noise trials, the lower limit of the one contraction was established in the way just described, and the lower limit of the other required contraction was $6 + 4.5 = 10.5$ µV/s higher than the individual minimum. The critical relaxation level the subject had to arrive at between the two contractions of a trial was 3 µV/s higher than the individual minimum. After the two contractions of a trial, the subject was always asked to judge whether the contractions differed or not on the following four-point rating scale:

1 = certain—no difference between the two contractions
2 = uncertain—no difference between the two contractions
3 = uncertain—difference between the two contractions
4 = certain—difference between the two contractions.

During the relaxation exercises and the assesment of the individual minimum, the subject sat in a comfortable chair and looked straight at the wall. During the

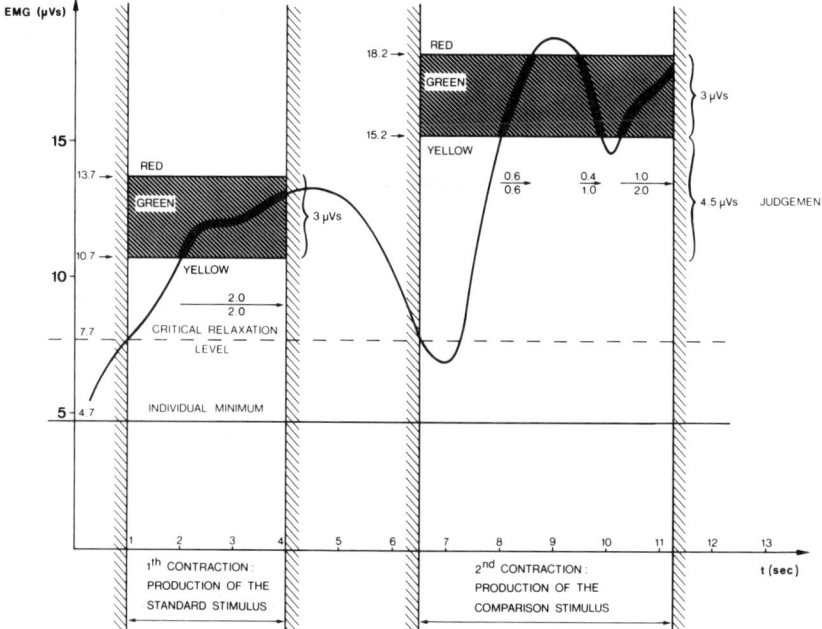

Figure 2. One possible trial of the signal detection experiment: Signal + noise.

signal detection trials the subject sat in front of a monitor with this chair. There was a small box fixed upon the monitor with a yellow (left), a green (middle), and a red (right) light. On the table in front of the monitor a second box was situated with four numbered push-buttons for the judgments of the subject.

The whole presentation of the trials was controlled automatically. The subjects received the instructions from the monitor. At the beginning of a trial they were instructed to relax the frontal muscle. It was attested from the screen when this was sufficiently attained—when muscle activity remained under the critical relaxation level. Then, the monitor gave the instruction to contract the frontal muscle for the first time while observing the lights. The meaning of the lights was explained on the screen. The subject contracted his frontal muscle by raising the eyebrows and "produced" green. At the end of the presentation time, the lights went off and the screen showed the instruction to relax. Having arrived at the critical relaxation level, the subject was instructed by the monitor to contract the frontal muscle for a second time. Following the second contraction, the screen showed the rating categories and their meaning as well as the request to make a judgement. The next trial began immediately after pressing the push-button—with the instruction to relax the frontal muscle. At the end of every 20 trials the program stopped. The monitor instructed the subject to take a short break. The subject finished the break by pressing a key.

At the beginning of the experiment the experimenter explained the trial structure in detail to the subject, and during the first trials again checked that the subject absolved the tasks correctly. Then the experimenter retired within earshot into the adjoining room.

Apparatus

EMG measures were obtained from the frontal muscle using Hellige surface electrodes (within diameter 10 mm). The horizontal lead position and application followed the recommendations of Zipp (1982). The electrodes were connected to a preamplifier which was fixed at the subject's shoulder. The preamplified signal was fed into a EMG amplifier (Zak, Simbach, FRG), then filtered with a 5.5—300 Hz bandpass filter, rectified and smoothed by a RC-filter (time constant $\tau = 25$ ms). An AD-converter of an R10 computer (Siemens, Stuttgart, FRG) transferred the analogue signal to digital values. The computer gave instructions to the subject in a dialogical manner, it turned on the lights, and registered the ratings of the subject.

Measurement Assumptions of the Procedure

An important prerequisite for the suitability of optical feedback in presenting the stimuli is the reliability and validity of the surface EMG (SEMG). Considering the relevant empirical results, we can take it for granted that the SEMG is a valid indicator of both the contraction level of the m. frontalis and the corollary discharges of the motor commands producing the contraction level. The SEMG registers fluctuations of the electrical potentials which take place at the membranes of the muscle fibers and which arrive at the skin surface passing the connective tissue (cf. Sauermann, 1986, for further details). The electrical potential depends on the innervation of motor units. The frequency of innervation and the number of motor units in action reflect the intensity of the motor command which is directly transmitted to the sensory cortex by corollary discharges (McCloskey, Gandevia, Potter, & Colebatch, 1983). On the other hand, there is a strict relationship between the number of motor units in action (recruitment), the frequency of innervation, and the force of muscle contraction (Schmidt, 1985; Desmedt, 1983). The intraindividual correlations between SEMG and short time force production vary from 0.93 to 0.99 (Lippold, 1952). Nevertheless, it has to be considered that the force of contraction—the frequency of innervation (the SEMG) being equally high—diminishes with continued contraction. Another way to describe this so-called effort effect is as follows: With increasing time, it costs more and more effort (requires more and more motor commands) to keep constant a defined force of contraction (Jones & Hunter, 1983). However, the effort effect only takes place in contractions exceeding 15% of the maximum force of the muscle, and here as well not within the first seconds (Laurig, 1970). Therefore, it will not occur in our experiment. Muscle tensions to be produced in the experimental trials always remain beneath 25 µV/s—the average maximum level of the frontal muscle is 161 µV/s (Bischoff, 1989)—and the single contractions rarely take longer than 3 seconds because it is quite easy for the subjects to keep their muscle tension within the green interval.

Characteristics of the Experimental Task Influencing Tension Perception

There are three characteristics of the experimental task which possibly modify the perceptual process but cannot be held constant:

- the subject's individual minimum of frontal muscle tension;
- the subject's capacity to regulate muscle tension so that the green light is on without interruption during signal presentation;
- the subject's capacity to relax the frontal muscle between the two contractions of a trial.

It is reasonable to assume that the perceptual performance will be better, the lower the minimal frontal muscle tension is, the better the subject is able to keep the green light continuously on, and the faster the subject relaxes between the contractions of a trial (Bischoff, 1989). We operationalized the three factors with suitable measures (see below) in order to control their influence with statistical methods.

Intraindividual Indices

The following intraindividual indices were computed:

P(A):   Sensibility of subject for muscle tension differences. This is a nonparametric index for the perceptual capacity, defined as the area beneath the individual's ROC-curve which characterizes the probability of hits as compared to false alarms. P(A) varies between 0.50 and 1.00. Because the distribution of P(A) has a tendency to be negatively skewed, P(A)-values were transformed into $2 \arcsin \sqrt{P(A)}$-values (McNicol, 1972). For group statistics we always used these transformed values.

P(A)-values were determined with the computer program "Signal Detection Rating Scale Program" by Dorfman and Alf (1972) in the revised version by Dorfman and Nelson resp. Harvey and Bashinsky.

B: Response bias of subject to use a lax vs. strong criterion when comparing muscle tensions. This nonparametric index is defined as the rating scale category at which the subject is equally disposed to signal and noise responses; mathematically speaking, at which P(S/s) + P(S/n) = 1. A small B-value indicates a strong criterion, that is, the subject has a tendency to judge the two contractions of a trial as equally high irrespective of their actual equality or difference (McNicol, 1972).

PUR: Percentage of uncertain responses, i.e., percentage of responses of categories 2 and 3. This index operationalizes the subject's response bias to judge cautious vs. decided irrespective of the true equality or difference between the contractions of a trial.

EMGmin: Minimal frontal muscle tension of the subject. The minimum is defined as median of the 10 1-second EMG integrals of the registration following the relaxation exercises.

FLG: Mean frequency of leaving the green interval during a single contraction. FLG is an index of the subject's capability to control the frontal muscle tension within the green interval.

RT: Mean recovery time between the two contractions of a trial. The recovery time is defined as the time between the end of the first contraction of a trial and moment of arriving at the critical relaxation level of the subject. RT operationalizes the subject's capability to relax the frontal muscle between the two contractions.

Reliability and Validity of the Signal Detection Design

The described indices, above all P(A), proved to be consistent and test-retest reliable within a six-week interval. They also meet important validity criterions: P(A) and B are statistically independent. Moreover, the sensitivity for differences of muscle tension is higher with respect to low tension levels than with high tension levels. This result reflects Weber-Fechner's psychophysical law, which obviously holds true for muscle tension perception as well (Bischoff, 1989).

Using this signal detection design we operationalize the hypotheses concerning the perceptual deficit of individuals suffering from myogenic headache as follows:

Individuals suffering from myogenic headache
1) smaller B-values, and
2) have smaller P(A)-values,
3) higher percentages of "uncertain"-responses than pain-free controls and migraineurs.

Results

For statistical analyses we used the computer programs P2V and P8D of BMDP (Dixon et al., 1983).

Sensibility P(A)

Table 1 shows the results of the one-way ANOVA with experimental groups as independant and transformed P(A) as dependant variable. For the sake of clearness, the transformation of P(A) was reversed.

Experimental groups differ in the postulated direction. Individuals suffering from myogenic headache exhibit, compared to migraineurs and pain-free controls, a diminished perceptual sensibility. These findings crystallize yet more clearly when we look at the linear contrast between the mean sensibility of the myogenic headache group and the averaged mean of the two other groups. The probability of the observed linear contrast—H0 being valid—is less or equal to .03.

As expected, the subjects' sensitivity correlates negatively with their EMGmin ($r = -0.23$; n.s.), FLG ($r = -0.42$; $p < 0.01$), and RT ($r = -0.35$; $p < 0.05$). The three task immanent parameters EMGmin, FLG, and RT do not covary with the experimental groups. Analysis of variance results in probabilities of $p < 0.28$ (EMGmin), $p < 0.68$ (FLG), and $p < 0.34$ (RT) that the group differences come about by chance. Therefore, they are not responsible for the group differences regarding P(A).

Table 1. ANOVA of P(A), B, and PUR.

	Myogenic Headache (N = 12)	Migraine (N = 15)	Normals (N = 12)	F (df = 2;36)	$p \leq$
P(A)	$\bar{x}_1 = 0.74$	$\bar{x}_2 = 0.88$	$\bar{x}_3 = 0.84$	3.27	.05
B	$\bar{x}_1 = 2.50$	$\bar{x}_2 = 2.52$	$\bar{x}_3 = 2.22$	2.39	.11
PUR	$\bar{x}_1 = 65.60$	$\bar{x}_2 = 52.70$	$\bar{x}_3 = 55.40$	3.40	.05

Response Biases B and PUR

ANOVA of B does not confirm the hypothesis (see Table 1). Contrary to our expectations, mean B of myogenic headache sufferers even exceeds mean B of the pain-free controls, indicating that myogenic headache sufferers use a laxer criterion than controls. But this is true for migraineurs, too. The linear contrast comparing all headache subjects and controls is statistically significant ($p < 0.05$).

The results regarding PUR is quite in line with the corresponding hypothesis. Individuals suffering from myogenic headache have a clearly higher percentage of "uncertain"-responses than migraineurs and pain-free controls (see Table 1). Comparing the myogenic headache group and the other groups combined by computing a linear contrast leads to p = 0.03.

PUR and P(A) correlate significantly with r = −0.50. It is not sensible to assume that the tendency to use "uncertain"-responses affects the perceptual capacity. The opposite is more probable. Individuals with reduced sensitivity will be aware of this fact to a certain degree and judge more cautiously for this reason. There is no longer a group difference regarding PUR in the analysis of covariance with P(A) as covariate. Even the linear contrast is compatible with H0, now (p = 0.09). That is, if the decreased P(A) of the myogenic headache sufferers is responsible for their tendency to use the "uncertain"-categories, then this is sufficient explanation for the group differences regarding PUR.

PUR and B correlate significantly with r = 0.47. Individuals judging cautiously have a laxer criterion. In our case, this "laxer" criterion of the myogenic headache sufferers coincides with the scale point 2.5, which is the point of undecidedness. B has about the same value in migraineurs (2.52). But this result must have been accomplished in another way than in myogenic headache sufferers, namely, by the migraineurs' more frequent use of the extreme categories 1 and 4.

Discussion

The experimental data corroborate the perceptual deficit hypothesis in important aspects. Individuals suffering from myogenic headache are less sensitive to voluntarily produced small muscle contractions and are, probably as a consequence of the reduced sensitivity, more cautious than pain-free controls and migraineurs when comparing muscle tensions.

The assumption that myogenic headache sufferers use stronger criterions than control groups was not confirmed. In interpreting this result we must take into account that B and PUR are mathematically coupled. The correlation between the two measures depends on the mean and the variance of the ratings in the total sample. For instance, if the ratings vary between the categories 1 and 2, then the cautious rater will get a laxer criterion than the determined. However, the more cautious rater will have the stronger criterion when the ratings distribute among the categories 3 and 4.

The (compared with the pain-free controls) lax criterions B of both headache groups must be equal for different reasons. In myogenic headache sufferers, they are lax because of the increased percentage of "uncertain"-responses, in migraineurs because of an increased percentage of responses belonging to category 4 ("certainly different"). The influence of PUR on B cannot be controlled by means of an analysis of covariance because the correlation between PUR and B differs in the particular experimental groups. The regression coefficients between dependant variable and covariate are not homogeneous. However, homogeneity is a prerequisite for the application of covariance analysis.

For us, the interpretation seems to be most sensible that in myogenic headache sufferers the tendency to judge cautiously dominates the bias to apply a strong criterion, i.e., to expect no differences between muscle tensions.

It remains questionable whether the results concerning the sensitivity deficit and the cautiousness can be generalized to reflex and tonic contractions. Probably, perception of reflex contractions is more difficult in general because in reflex contractions the individual lacks the information of corrolary discharges. Similarily, we cannot be sure that the results are valid for the activity of other muscles than the frontal muscle, too.

Migraineurs do not differ from normals with respect both to sensitivity and judgemental decidedness. This implicates that the perceptual deficit is typical of individuals suffering from myogenic headache. In addition, this means the deficient sensitivity cannot be interpreted as a consequence of the pain disorder. The assumption that chronic pain—irrespective of its origin—impairs the perceptual capacities should be true for migraineurs as well. Nevertheless, the experiment prevents one from determining whether the perceptual deficit is a cause or a concomitant symptom of myogenic headache, and whether it develops on a constitutional basis or as a consequence of learning.

We propose an explanation which interprets both, the etiology of myogenic headache and of the perceptual deficit, within the framework of the same model.

Our causal scheme (Bischoff & Traue, 1983) postulates that myogenic headache is caused by dysfunctional activity of head and neck muscles. Muscle activities are dysfunctional when they lead to a reduced blood supply of the muscles used, with the consequence that pain substances are released affecting the thresholds of mechanical and biochemical nociceptors (Mense & Schmidt, 1977; Mense, 1981). The psychophysiological basis of dysfunctional muscle activity are the functions of the motor system. Muscle activity is the physiological correlative of motor acts: movements and postures. Motor acts are voluntary acts, i.e., instrumental behaviors, or unvoluntary acts, i.e., reflex, instinctive, or emotional behaviors. Voluntary motor acts may be modified by operant conditioning, involuntary motor acts by classical conditioning. Dysfunctional muscle activity develops from conditioned motor acts requiring this activity. In myogenic headache, two behavioral fields seem to be relevant in which these conditioning processes take place:
1) expression of emotions and states of general arousal;
2) physical and mental exertion accompanied by static activity of head and neck muscles.

ad 1): Dysfunctional muscle activity develops when the individual is punished for the expression of emotions or states of general arousal so that he learns to inhibit expressive behavior. Experimental studies of our research group (Traue, Gottwald, Henderson, & Bakal, 1985a; Traue, Mahoney, & Bischoff, 1985b;

Bischoff & Sauermann, 1985) show that compared to controls myogenic headache sufferers have a reduced expressiveness in emotional and generally activating situations, paralleled by increased muscle activity. We assume that dysfunctional muscle activity develops in these cases because there is no overt behavior "consuming" the energy of involuntary motor impulses. Simultaneously, inhibitory motor programs start working. They again result in motor impulses.

The perception of muscle tension is not only a response but one of the discriminative stimuli for the experience and expression of emotion (Laird, 1984; Zajonc & Markus, 1984). Following the laws of behavior, chaining perception will be inhibited or extinguished when the expression of emotion is inhibited. In addition, we expect that the intensity of the emotional experience diminishes, and that the individual is less capable to decode the quality of the emotion in question.

ad 2): Dysfunctional muscle activity develops when the individual is positively or negatively reinforced for physical or intellectual exertion. That mainly holds for exertion accompanied by static activitiy of the head and neck muscles, because the oxygen supply of muscles becomes insufficient very quickly when static in contrast to dynamic muscle activity is needed (Ulmer, 1985). Myogenic headache has a remarkable prevalence in certain professions: in secretaries, pianists, workers in front of a computer screen or at a desk (Robinson, 1980). These persons engage in activities which, as result of the arm position or of involuntary reactions to cognitive involvement, require static work of the shoulder, neck, and head muscles. On the other hand, a very strong achievement motivation and an extreme fear of failure is often typical of mygenic headache patients (Passchier, v.d. Helm-Hylkema, & Orlebeke, 1984). Positive or negative reinforcement of work done which is realized by means of operant motor acts leads to dysfunctional muscle effort when the operant motor acts are excessively practiced as a result of this reinforcement. In this connection, it is of special interest that an increased tonic level of the muscles enhances the efficiency of responses. Reaction times become shorter, tasks requiring visual discrimination can be solved better (Moran & Cleary, 1984), cognitive processes and problem solving are facilitated (Jacobson, 1973; McGuigan, 1978). That is, muscle activity can be conditioned quite directly when achievement behavior is reinforced.

The perception of muscle tension is extinguished when the individual excessively practices operant motor and intellectual behaviors. It loses its original function as a discriminative or triggering stop stimulus. Simultaneously, we expect that the perceived intensity of the effort to which the excessive behavior is combined declines.

Meanwhile, there is encouraging empirical support for the causal scheme of myogenic headache and the etiology of the perceptual deficit, though many of its implications still need closer examination. In the present context, a finding of Schlote (in this volume) is worthy of notice: Office-workers complaining of myogenic headache exhibit significantly higher muscle tension levels throughout their working day, but in spite of it, they feel less stressed than their pain-free colleagues doing the same work! This result may be interpreted in terms of the postulated effect of the perceptual deficit: Punished or extinguished perception of muscle tension reduces not only the sensitivity and decidedness of tension perception but, as a consequence, the perceived intensity of effort, too.

References

Appelbaum, K.A., Blanchard, E.B. & Andrasik, F. (1984). Muscle discrimination ability at three muscle sites in three headache groups. *Biofeedback & Self-Regulation, 9,* 421—430.
Birbaumer, N. (1975). *Physiologische Psychologie.* Berlin: Springer-Verlag.
Bischoff, C. (1989). *Wahrnehmung von Muskelspannung. Eine signalentdeckungstheoretische Analyse bei Personen mit Muskelkontraktionskopfschmerz.* Göttingen: Hogrefe.
Bischoff, C., & Sauermann, G. (1985). Nicht-instrumentelles motorisches Verhalten von Personen mit und ohne Spannungskopfschmerz. In H.-U. Wittchen & J.C. Brengelmann (Eds.), *Psychologische Therapie bei chronischen Schmerzpatienten* (pp. 93—111). Berlin: Springer-Verlag.
Bischoff, C., & Traue, H.C. (1983). Myogenic headache. In K. Holroyd, B. Schlote, & H. Zenz (Eds.), *Perspectives in research on headache* (pp. 66—90). Toronto/Lewiston, NY: C.J. Hogrefe.
Blanchard, E.B., Jurish, S.E., Andrasik, F., & Epstein, L.H. (1981). The relationship between muscle discrimination ability and response to relaxation training in three kinds of headache. *Biofeedback and Self-Regulation, 6,* 537—545.
Desmedt, J.E. (1983). Size principle of motoneuron recruitment and the calibration of muscle force and speed in man. In J.E. Desmedt (Ed.), *Motor control mechanisms in health and disease.* New York: Raven Press.
Dixon, W.J., Brown, M.B., Engelman, L., Frane, J.W., Hill, M.A., Jennrich, R.I., & Toborek, J.B. (1983). *BMDP Statistical Software.* Berkeley: University of California Press.
Dorfman, D.D., & Alf, E. (1972). *Signal detection rating-scale method program.* (Modified by Beavers, L., 1972, latest revisions by Dorfman, D.D., & Nelson, K., modified for CDC 6400 by Harvey, L.O., & Bashinski, H.S.) Boulder: University of Colorado Press.
Dorfman, D.D, & Alf, E., Jr. (1968). Maximum-likelihood estimation of parameters of signal-detection theory and determination of confidence intervals-rating method data. *Journal of Mathematical Psychology, 6,* 487—496.
Epstein, L.H., & Cinciripini, P.M. (1981). Behavioral control of tension headaches. In J.M. Ferguson & C.B. Taylor (Eds.), *The comprehensive handbook of behavioral medicine, Vol. 2.* Jamaica: Spectrum Press.
Fordyce, W. (1976). *Behavioral methods for chronic pain and illness.* St. Louis, MO: Mosby.
Fowler, R.S., & Kraft, G.H. (1974). Tension perception in patients having pain associated with chronic muscle tension. *Archives of Physical and Medical Rehabilitation, 55,* 28—30.
Jacobson, E. (1973). Electrophysiology of mental activities and introduction to the psychological process of thinking. In F.J. McGuigan & R.A. Schoonover (Eds.), *The psychophysiology of thinking* (pp. 3—31). New York: Academic Press.
Jacobson, E. (1983). *Progressive relaxation.* Chicago: University of Chicago Press.
Jones, L.A., & Hunter, J.W. (1983). Force and EWG correlates of constant effort contractions. *European Journal of Applied Physiology, 51,* 75—83.
Laird, J.D. (1984). The real role of facial response in the experience of emotion: A reply to Tourangeau and Ellsworth, and others. *Journal of Personality and Social Psychology, 47,* 909—917.

Laurig, W. (1970). *Elektromyographie als arbeitswissenschaftliche Untersuchungsmethode von statischer Muskelarbeit.* Berlin: Beutz-Vertrieb GmbH.

Lippold, O.C.J. (1952). The relation between integrated action potentials in a human muscle and its isometric tension. *Journal of Physiology, 117,* 492—499.

McCloskey, D.I., Gandevia, S., Potter, E.K., & Colebatch, J.G. (1983). Muscle sense and effort: Motor commands and judgement about muscular contraction. In J.E. Desmedt (Ed.) *Advances in neurology, Vol. 39: Motor control mechanisms in health and disease* (pp. 151—167). Bethesda, MD: American Physiological Society.

McGuigan, F.J. (1978). Imagery and thinking: Covert functioning of motor system. In G.E. Schwartz & D. Shapiro (Eds.), *Consciousness and self-regulation, Vol. 2.* New York: Plenum.

McNicol, D. (1972). *A primer of signal detection theory.* London: Allen & Unwin.

Mense, S. (1981). Sensibilisation of groups IV muscle receptors to bradykinin by 5-hydroxytryptamine and prostaglendine E2. *Brain Research, 225,* 95—105.

Mense, S., & Schmidt, R.F. (1977). Muscle pain: Which receptors are responsible for the transmission of noxious stimuli? In F.C. Rose (Ed.), *Physiological aspects of clinical neurology.* Oxford: Blackwell.

Moran, C.C., & Cleary, P.J. (1984). Some benefits of high frontalis tension in tension headache sufferers. *Headache, 24,* 331—338.

Passchier, J.H., v.d. Helm-Hylkema, H., & Orlebeke, J.F. (1976). Personality and headache type: A controlled study. *Headache, 16,* 20—23.

Pikoff, H. (1984). Is the muscular model of headache still viable? A review of conflicting data. *Headache, 24,* 186—198.

Robinson, C.A. (1980). Cervical spondylosis and muscle contraction headaches. In D.J. Dalessio (Ed.), *Wolff's headache and other head pain.* New York: Oxford University Press.

Sauermann, G. (1986). *Elektromyographie als psychophysiologische Methode.* Dissertation, Universität Ulm.

Schmidt, R.F. (1985). Motorische Systeme. In R.F. Schmidt & G. Thews (Eds.), *Physiologie des Menschen* (pp. 87—118). Berlin: Springer-Verlag.

Stevens, S.S. (1975). *Psychophysics: Introduction to its perceptual, neural and social prospects.* New York: Wiley.

Stilson, D.W., Matus, J., & Ball, G.S. (1980). Relaxation and subjective estimates of muscle tension: Implications for a central effort theory of muscle control. *Biofeedback and Self-Regulation, 5,* 19—36.

Traue, H.C., Gottwald, A., Henderson, P.R., & Bakal, D.A. (1985a). Nonverbal expressiveness and activity in tension headache sufferers and controls. *Journal of Psychosomatic Research, 29,* 375—381.

Traue, H.C., Mahoney, A.M., & Bischoff, C. (1985b). Toward a new understanding of tension headache. In D. Papakostopoulos, S. Butler, & I. Martin (Eds.), *Clinical and experimental neuropsychophysiology* (pp. 558—577). London: Croom Helm.

Ulmer, H.V. (1985). Arbeitsphysiologie—Umweltphysiologie. In R.F. Schmidt, & G. Thews (Eds.), *Physiologie des Menschen* (pp. 602—627). Berlin: Springer-Verlag.

Wolf-Cramer, B. (1984). Zum Problem der Diagnostik des Spannungskopfschmerzes. *Psychotherapie, Psychosomatik, Medizinische Psychologie, 34,* 81—89.

Zajonc, R.B., & Markus, H. (1984). Affect and cognition: The hard interface. In C.E. Izard, J. Kagan, & R.B. Zajonc (Eds.), *Emotions, cognition and behavior* (pp. 73—102). Cambridge: Cambridge University Press.

Zipp, P. (1982). Recommendations for the standardization of lead positions in surface electromyography. *European Journal of Applied Physiology, 50,* 41—54.

Behavioral Inhibition in Stress Disorders and Myogenic Pain

Harald C. Traue

This chapter reviews the role of inhibitory mechanisms in stress disorders. It is intended to draw attention to the fact that there is considerable evidence of an inverse relationship between overt nonverbal expressiveness and physiologic activity. Inhibition considered as an active process in the individual must be included among those mechanisms of social, emotional, and behavior regulations that are responsible for the etiology and maintainence of several psychophysiological disorders.

Results from experimental headache research support the general hypothesis concerning the inverse relationship between expressiveness and physiological activity. Muscle contraction headache patients and normal pain-free controls were confronted with a social stressor while muscle tension and their interactional behavior were recorded. The headache groups showed greater muscle activation and less nonverbal expressiveness in response to stress. The data analysis for the total sample showed negative correlations between EMG scores and expressiveness ratings. Finally, this chapter includes behavioral data from clinical interviews. Nonverbal expressiveness ratings were correlated with social support scales. The results demonstrated a significant relationship between expressiveness change scores and social support. The more expressive individuals are, the better do they judge their social support system.

In 1937, H.G. Wolff and his colleagues observed that headache sufferers were often nonexpressive individuals characterized by "a quality of studied poise, most often accompanied with tense facial expression with furrowed forehead, contraction between the eyebrows, quick moving eyes and perhaps uneasy laughter" (p. 905). He later noted that sustained muscle contraction activity in the head and neck regions was also characteristic of headache sufferers (Tunis & Wolff, 1954). Although after some decades of headache research one would not expect to find all these patients to be unexpressive and tense, the relationship between inhibition of expressive behavior and its physiological counterparts still forms the center of interest not only for pain patients, but for psychophysiological or so-called stress disorders in general.

An understanding of the relationship between behavioral inhibition and arousal can add substantial knowledge about an important mechanism in the etiology and maintenance of psychophysiological disorders. Although there is general agreement among researchers and clinicians that psychophysiological disorders are mediated by social and psychological factors, and that these illnesses are exacerbated by emotional states, "psychosomatic medicine must eventually seek to explain how psychosocial stimuli are translated into acute or chronic changes in structure and in physiological and biochemical function" (Weiner, 1977).

This paper addresses the role of behavioral inhibition and increased physiological reactivity as part of maladaption in the interaction between an individual and his or her social environment. Although reduced expressiveness and heightened bodily reactions may be adaptive when faced with a social stress situation, in the long run these behaviors can take a harmful toll on the organism. As Engel (1986, p. 472) puts it: "The risk of being given an opportunity to develop adaptability in response to acute challenges is that the adaptations may not serve long-range goals very well."

Emotion, Stress and Illness

Recent conceptualizations view emotion as a process of appraisal of transactions with the environment (Lazarus, 1966). Emotions are believed to comprise a variety of components: cognitive interpretation of intero- and exteroceptive stimuli, physiological pattern of arousal, motoric mobilization, affective experience, and behavioral expressions. These different components are mediated by the central nervous system as result of the interaction between the individual and the social and physical environment. The emotion can be considered as a response to environmental stimuli or as an act to control the environment.

Brady (1975) makes a basic distinction between emotional events that occur "inside" and "outside" the skin. Thus, cognitive, experimental and most of the physiological processes that are within the skin are covert events, while verbal and motor behavior are overt events. Expressive motor behavior in emotion has two important functions: First, as a communicative function, this behavior facilitates regulation of person-environment transactions; and second, the feedback function of behavioral expression controls the internal (intraindividual) regulation of emotion. Active responding may influence the experienced stress indirectly through the attenuation of the stressful agent (controlling the environment), or directly through self-regulation. Thus, expressive behavior is simultaneously part of emotion processes and a coping response.

Reduced Expressiveness in Psychophysiological Disorders

Recently it has been recognized that there is considerable variability among individuals in terms of expressive behavior. Individuals who appear inhibited in either verbal or motor responses toward emotional stimuli have been labelled "internalized" (Buck, 1979; Jones, 1935), "alexithymic" (Sifneos, 1973), or "repressed" (Byrne, 1961). It is generally assumed that the inability to express emotion or the inhibition of that expression represents poor coping with one's environment. Expressive behavior is of interest to researchers in psychosomatic medicine because of its relationship to physiological activity. There is considerable evidence from empirical studies showing a consistently inverse relationship between overt expressions of emotion and autonomic activity. Because it is believed that elevated activity in a particular physiological system may increase a person's vulnerability to develop a psychosomatic disorder in that system, factors that contribute to physiological reactivity are important to the understanding of the etiology and maintenance of such disorders.

Early clinical accounts of psychosomatic patients revealed that these individuals frequently complain of an inability or inhibition of direct emotional expression in their social environment. Ruesch (1948) described psychosomatic patients as displaying inappropriate social communication. Stokvis (1953) reported that repressed aggressive feelings were common in patients suffering from psychosomatic disorders. Wittkower and Lipowski (1966) suggested that the relatively high incidence of psychosomatic complaints in Kuwaiti women may be the result of the limited freedoms for women in that society. In general, situations fostering emotional restraint were considered to have pathogenic qualities. In support of this Meissner (1977) described the family interaction of psychosomatic patients as highly disciplined in the expression of negative feelings. Similarily, parents of children with somatic conversion reactions were found to be verbally inhibited on the topic of sexuality. Gannon (1981) observed in her work with the Peace Corps that those volunteers who adopted a passive strategy to cope with stress in a third-world country developed more gastro-intestinal problems than those who responded behaviorally to the stressors.

Many of the above reports are based on anecdotal evidence and lack an empirical foundation. Yet they were important, for they determined the direction of contemporary experimental work in clinical psychology and behavioral medicine. Recently, Buck (1979) hypothesized that without behavioral expression of emotion, internal emotional activity is said to be intensified. A series of experiments carried out by Buck and his colleagues have demonstrated a negative relationship between expressive behavior and autonomic activity such as GSR and heart rate. Persons who displayed overt manifestations of emotion were found to have lower physiological reactions in response to emotional stimuli than persons who were less expressive. Buck concluded that continual increased physiological responding may be maladaptive in the long run and exert a physical toll on the organism.

According to Sternbach (1971) the emotion most likely to be associated with psychosomatic illness is anger. The relationship of anger to physiological reactivity and behavioral suppression in social situations has been studied experimentally. Hokanson and Burgess (1962) demonstrated that direct aggression toward an anger-provoking person had the effect of returning elevated systolic blood pressure to resting levels much faster than when aggression was not allowed. Gambaro and Rabin (1969) compared decreases in diastolic blood pressure as function of permissible and impermissible expression of anger and the more or less guilt-loaded personality. Their analysis of variance showed a main effect for a blood pressure reduction based on the permission of anger expression as well as for the low guilt-loaded personality.

More recently, differences in expressive behavior between groups suffering from psychosomatic disorders and normals have been investigated with experimental designs. Hollaender and Florin (1983) examined expression of emotion and peak expiratory flow rate (PEFR) in 14 asthmatic children and controls during a competitive achievement task. The asthmatics were found to be significantly less expressive as measured by frequency and duration of facial signs than the normal children. Furthermore, duration of expressed emotion showed a significant negative correlation with PEFR. In another study, Florin, Freudenberg, and Hollaender (1985) replicated the findings that asthmatic children were less expressive than normals, but that this difference held only for negative emotions. Differences between groups were observed during a stress-inducing task but not during a joy-inducing one.

Anderson (1981) examined the relationship between the verbal expression of affect and stress in relation to physiological responses in a variety of psychosomatic disorders. Patients with tension and migraine headaches, rheumatoid arthritis, or hypertension were compared to normals during stress and recovery periods. The results of this study supported the hypothesized negative relationship between verbal expressions of emotions and physiological responses. However, this relationship was observed for all subjects and not specifically for the psychosomatic groups. Though the negative relationships were weakest in the normal subjects and highest in the pain groups, they were not significantly different from those observed in the other groups.

In a recent study, Malatesta, Jonas, and Izard (1987) suggested that suppressed emotion—specifically suppressed facial signs of emotion—might he associated with illness and the reporting of physical symptoms. The study examined this relationship under conditions of emotional arousal. Healthy adult women underwent emotion-inducing procedures for anger, anxiety and sadness, and were videotaped while describing their emotional reactions. Correlational statistics indicated that physical symptoms were almost exclusively negatively correlated with emotion expression. In summarizing their results, one can note that mainly the sum skin score and the sum arthritis score were negatively correlated, while the coronary/circulatory latency sum score was not significantly correlated with the emotional expressiveness patterns.

Expressiveness Training and Its Effects

For the most part, a relationship between the reduced behavioral output and increased physiological reactivity to emotional stimuli has been supported. Moreover, psychosomatic patients appear to be less expressive and more physiologically reactive than normals. If behavioral suppression is an important factor in psychophysiological disorders, then therapeutic interventions training the appropriate skills in expression of emotion should be effective. Indeed, there is some evidence to support this conclusion. One early psychodynamically oriented study reported the effects of learned overt emotional expression in skin disorder patients (Seitz, 1953). Patients were encouraged to express hostile feelings during the interviews with the therapist, but to refrain from aggressive actions outside of the treatment setting. Nearly half of the patients disobeyed these instructions and showed greater improvement than those who complied with the therapists instructions. Seitz concluded that paradoxical injunction promoted the expression of emotion which in turn contributed to improved symptom improvement.

Katz, Wittkower, Vavruska, Telner, and Ferguson (1957) subjected eczema patients to interviews designed to provide a release or discharge for aggressive feelings. They noted that this strategy reduced eczema symptoms. Furthermore, when they divided those patients who where relatively free in emotional expression and those who were not, they could accurately predict their reactions to histamine injections. Nine out of the twelve expressive patients showed a flare-up to the injection (which is the healthy reaction) while six of the seven nonexpressive patients did not show the functional flare-up reaction.

Emotional skills training has also proved beneficial in the treatment of duodenal ulcers. Brooks and Richardson (1980) described a tendency among ulcer patients to inhibit displays of negative emotion, to be conformative, resentful, frustrated, and non-assertive. They targeted this constellation of characteristics in a treatment study of ulcer patients. Patients first received four sessions of anxiety management training including restructuring of irrational beliefs, replacement of negative self-statements, and progressive relaxation. Patients then received four sessions of assertiveness training during which they were encouraged to learn prudent self-expression and to replace feelings of chronic resentment. Patients were asked to exercise and test the assertive behaviors at home and at work. The treatment groups reported significant reductions in anxiety, ulcer pain, and drug consumption. These reductions were not found in a matched control group. Most impressive were the results of the 3-year follow-up in this study. Only one out of the nine persons in the treatment group suffered a relapse, while more than half of the control group experienced relapses.

Social Stress and Myogenic Pain

Dysfunctional muscular activity is increasingly being recognized as an etiological and susceptibility factor in various myogenic pain disorders like muscle contraction headache, low back pain, myofascial pain syndrom, bruxism, temporomandibular joint disfunction, and some forms of rheumatic arthritis. The critical muscular activity may be classified as dysfunctional increase, prolonged recovery following stressful events, heightened tension in relief situations and prolonged duration of stressful situations. An individual develops myogenic pain in a particular muscular system when the muscle activity increases to a critical point within a certain period of time (Bischoff & Traue, 1983).

In addition to spatial-temporal coordination of voluntary and reflex-like movements and general organic variables, muscle activity patterns are part of emotional processes. The latter is mainly hyperactivated under social and personally relevant stressful encounter. These so-called social or natural stressors (Schwartz, 1983) are encountered on the job, or with family or peer group; they relate to interpersonal problems and are integrated into life style; and they tend to influence them over long time periods ranging from hours, weeks, or even months. The results of Traue, Bischoff and Zenz (1986), Flor, Turk, and Birbaumer (1985), and Schlote (1987) indicate that the experimental use of such social or long-term stressors in a laboratory or ambulantory assessment are successful in differentiating myogenic pain patients from controls in terms of increased and prolonged muscle tension.

If one considers muscle activity as part of more general pattern of human motor activity in emotion processes it is evident that muscle tension may be controlled by learning mechanisms. Classical or operant conditioning of motor behavior may lead to hyperactivity in a particular muscle system. Expressive behavior is prone to become punished under certain conditions of socialisation starting an individual history of increased tension and reduced expressiveness.

Reduced Expressiveness, Muscle Tension, and Social Stress

In order to test the hypothesis of an inverse relationship between muscle tension and nonverbal expressiveness we induced a social stressor situation (Traue, Gottwald, Henderson, & Bakal, 1985). We compared muscular reactivty and behavioral expressiveness data of a homogeneous group of young tension-headache sufferers with a matched group of pain-free controls. The clinical group consisted of 18 patients with a history of tension headache (weekly headache frequency was 1.6, mean intensity was 4.8 on a 7-point scale). The experimental procedure comprised a beginning relaxation treatment, and an interactive social stressor by presenting a TAT-picture with the instruction to prepare a story to be told later, telling the TAT-story, being criticized for the story by a confederate of the experimenter, and the final response of the subjects with respect of the whole situation (see Figure 1).

The EMG measures were obtained bilaterally from the frontalis and the right trapezius muscle. The EMG data within each of the experimental sequences were baseline adjusted and expressed as difference scores. The mean differences for all the stressors are summarized in Figure 2. There were no significant baseline differences in frontal muscle activity. The headache group evidenced significantly greater muscle activity in response to the social stress situation. This result corraborates an earlier experiment with a somewhat different stress situation (Traue, Bischoff, & Zenz, 1986).

Behavioral Inhibition in Stress Disorders and Myogenic Pain 35

Figure 1. Experimental design.

Physiological Measurement
EMG m. frontalis left
EMG m. frontalis right
EMG m. trapezius right

Behavioral Assessment
Head movement
Hand movement
Expressiveness
Tension
Activity

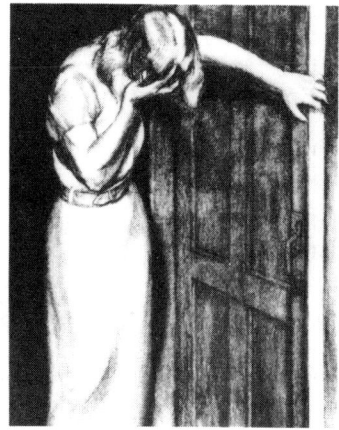

Relaxation Baseline Anticipation TAT-Story Critique Response

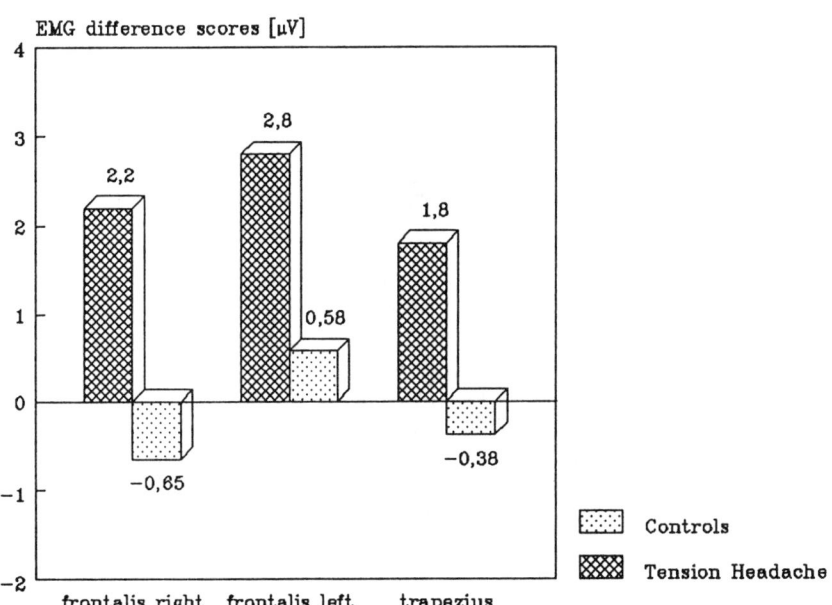

Figure 2. EMG difference scores collapsed over the total experimental stressor.

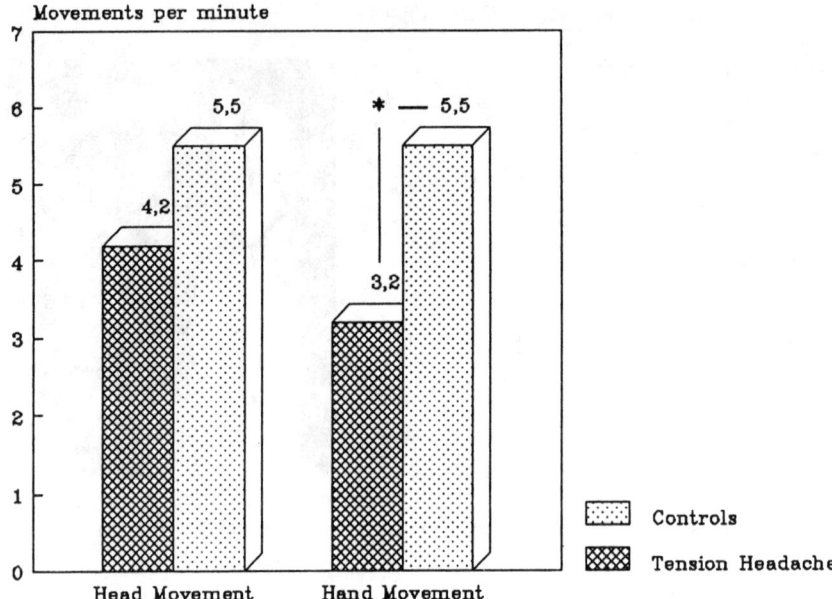

Figure 3. Number of head and hand movements collapsed over the total stress (* < .05).

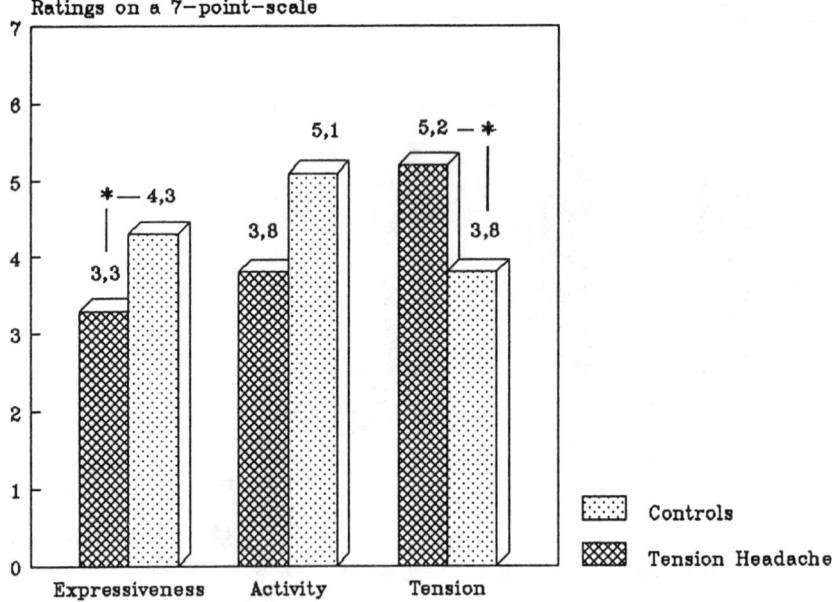

Figure 4. Ratings of facial behavior collapsed over the total stress (* < .05).

Three independent raters assessed five behavioral variables of expressiveness: head movement, hand movements, facial expressiveness, communicative activity, and facial tension. The last three variables were judged on seven-point Likert scales. Figures 3 and 4 summarize the behavioral data for the stress experiment. In general, the headache group displayed less head and hand movements during the stressful encounter; however, the differences were significant only at an early point of the whole stress sequence. As expected the headache subjects displayed significantly higher levels of facial tension. Comparison of the group means indicated significant differences in expressiveness and communicative activity. The headache group exhibited less facial activity.

The headache group differed from controls across the experimental stressor in terms of greater muscle tension, higher rated levels of facial tension, and reduced facial expressiveness. In order to assess the overall relationship between measures, product-moment correlations were calculated for subjects across both groups. Rated facial tension levels and actual EMG activity correlated positively. The nonverbal expressiveness and communicative activity consistently correlated negatively with muscle tension. Measures found to be of greatest value in discriminating groups tended to show the largest and most significant negatively correlated relationships with EMG activity. These findings demonstrate that, for example, individuals rated least expressive tended to display the greatest muscle tension.

The results of the present study add to the growing literature which suggest that "behavioral inhibition" is an active condition of the individual and may be reflective of personal coping styles characteristic for a subgroup of patients with stress disorders. Furthermore, this dynamics associated with behavioral inhibition/musculoskeletal activation need to be examined in the context of therapeutic intervention, especially in terms of providing patients with strategies and skills for increasing their awareness and expression of bodily feelings and emotions in social stress situations.

Reduced Expressiveness and Social Support

The findings in the former study support the hypothesis of an inverse relationship between expresssiveness and arousal reflecting a possible psychobiological connection between reduced expressiveness and the muscular activity in forehead and neck regions. If this inverse relationship occurs more likely under negative emotional stimulation, e.g., under particular stressful encounter in job or family, a deficit in nonverbal expressiveness may have related additional effects. If one interprets a reduced nonverbal expressiveness under social stressful encounters as a deficit in coping with these stressors, then nonexpressive individuals lack the ability to handle these stressors. Florin (1985) describes four different but related possibilities or reasons for inhibited expressiveness:

1. Reduced expressiveness can be used to avoid an active and stressful dispute that could help to clear a social situation.
2. Since emotional expressiveness is acutely associated with heightened arousal, reduced expressiveness can be used to avoid an individual's momentary arousal.
3. Previously expressive individuals might anticipate that people in the social surrounding could react with anxiety or anger if they express emotions, and such a situation could develop into an additional stressor.
4. An individual could be afraid of showing private information, which could increase the personal vulnerability of becoming emotionally harmed.

In coping with stressors, social support is known as a *protective system*. It is very probable, that nonverbal expressiveness as part of coping behavior also helps to maintain a social support system. There is overwhelming empirical evidence from social psychology that individual differences in nonverbal expressiveness correspond, for example, to helping behavior, the estimation of attractiveness, the reduction of interpersonal distance, and self-disclosing behavior of partners in conversation. All these behaviors are related to social support. Cobb (1976) defines social support as individual beliefs of being cared for, loved, estimated, valued, and belonging to a network of communication and mutual obligation. These beliefs protect individuals against the harmful influence of life events, daily hassles and other stressors. Pennebaker and Hoover (1986) showed the beneficial effects of simply talking about traumatic childhood events in adults: Adults who had not disclosed these traumatic events from the past to friends or relatives were more likely to report current health problems for a longer period of time.

To test the hypothesis of a positive relationship between expressiveness indicators and social support skills, we rated and coded several behavioral variables from interview data material of a group of chronic headache sufferers (Traue, in press). The clinical group consisted of 35 chronic headache patients including migraine, tension, and mixed headache (cf. Table 1).

Table 1. The group of chronic headache patients.

N = 35	(male = 13, female = 22)	
Mean age	41.70 years	
Range	16–69 years	
Headache since	18.23 years	(s = 13.39)
Mean intensity (10-Point-Scale)	7.11	(s = 1.30)
Weekly mean frequency	3.29	(s = 0.90)

With a mean pain duration of about 18 years, these patients are a typical group of chronic headache patients. The patients were referred to our outpatient pain clinic by other clinics or by physicians in private practice. As part of the pain clinic, the Department of Medical Psychology specializes in headache diagnosis and treatment. The patients come to the Department for several diagnostic procedures. Initially, the patients were interviewed with a semi-structured behavior analytical interview, which was also videotaped. From these tapes two 3-minute parts with the topics "behavior in recreation" and "behavior in sexuality" were selected. The latter is a more private and tabu topic, the former a more simple and easy-to-talk-about topic.

Table 2 shows a simplified listing of the applied rating and coding system, which is more elaborated than the nonverbal rating system from the earlier reported study.

Table 2. Simplified coding and rating scheme.

Head movements (frequency)
Hand-head-contact (duration, frequency)
Nervous mouth movements (duration frequency)
Speaking (duration frequency)
Eye contact (duration frequency)
Smiling (frequency)
Expressiveness (rating on a 7-point-scale)
Tension (rating on a 7-point-scale)
Nervousness (rating on a 7-point scale)

Social support variables were derived from a behaviorally oriented German personality questionnaire, the "Biographical Inventory for the Diagnosis of Behavior" (*Biographisches Inventar für Verhaltensstörungen;* Jäger, Lischer, Münster & Ritz, 1976). Some of the subscales of this particular inventory are very similar to social support scales, and they include items that are identical to those appearing in special social support scales. As indicators of social support we took the subscales: *Social Status, Social Activity, Parental Upbringing Behavior,* and *Extraversion* as an additional scale.

Following the coding and rating procedure of the interview behavior (described elsewhere, cf. Traue, in press) product-moment correlations between the behavioral data and the subjective social support scales were calculated. This resulted in two separate correlation tables, one from the data of the report of sexuality and one from the report of recreational behavior. Overall, however, these correlation coefficients were rather small. Therefore, the intraindividual differences between the expressive behaviors from the sexuality and recreation topics of the interviews were calculated and related to the questionnaire data. It was hypothesized that a decrease in expressiveness from the neutral theme to the tabu theme will result in additional information in respect of the individuals overt reaction to social stress. This procedure lead to a new matrix of correlation coefficients (see Table 3).

Table 3. Product-moment-correlations between behavior difference-scores (sexuality-recreation) and social support indices (df = 34, * = p<.05, ** = p<.01).

	Social stress	Parental upbringing behavior	Social activity		Extraversion
Head shaking	−.51**	−.03	−.36*		.04
Head movement (total)	−.39*	−.22	−.17	I	−.21
Expressiveness	−.03	−.29	−.29		−.08
Tension	.11	.17	.48**		−.09
Nervousness	−.19	.39*	.05	II	−.08
Nervous mouth movements	.23	−.09	.09		.03
Speech frequency	.16	−.06	.11		−.46
Speech duration	−.32*	.01	−.33*		−.01
Eye contact duration	−.15	−.15	−.54**	III	.00
Smiling frequency	.01	−.31*	−.38*		−.15

The relationship between the expressiveness data and the social support scales within the gained correlation table are somewhat complex and show several single significant and considerable large correlations. Space does not allow interpretation of these single relations, though in summarizing the results a more general explanation can be given.

First of all, it is necessary to know that small scores in the scales *Social Status, Social Activity* and *Parental Upbringing* indicate a good social support system. Secondly, the behavior data were structured as three partly independent factors by a factor analysis: (1) Expressiveness with head movements and expressiveness, (2) Tension with the ratings of tension, nervousness, nervous mouth movements and speech frequency, and (3) Activity with speech duration, eye contact and smiling.

The negative coefficients between the social support scales and the expressiveness behavior variables in Subtable I show this effect: The more expressive individuals were on the recreational topic, the better their scores on the social support scales. Moreover, the less expressive individuals were on the tabu topic *Sexuality*, the worse their social support scores. Subtable II shows positive correlations between tension and behavior ratings and the social support scales. The interpretation is quite similar to that one in Subtable I. Again Subtable III like subtable I shows similar relationships.

There is a very strong relationship between social activity and tension, as well as eye contact and smiling frequency. A high value in social activity is typical of individuals describing themselves as unable to make social contacts or maintain relationships to partners, and being inhibited in self-disclosing private information. The data demonstrate on the behavioral level not only that, but which reduction in nonverbal expressiveness is highly related to the social situation of the patient.

This study tested, independent of the particular headache type, the more social psychological hypothesis of a relation between overt expressive behavior and the subjective report of social support indicators. The data demonstrate that a decrease in expressiveness from a neutral relative to a tabu theme in terms of intraindividual differences are related to social support scales. This is the case although no or only minor correlations were found without looking for intraindividual differences. This result supports the notion that expressiveness as a coping style is more a state variable depending on the stressfulness of a particular situation than a trait variable. To this extent the data are in accordance with other experimental results like that from Florin, Freudenberg, and Hollaender (1985), who found inhibition of emotional expressiveness in their asthmatic children when negative emotions were induced by social stress, but not while their subjects where looking at a funny TV movie. Very similar are the data on muscle reactivity. Again muscle tension overactivity is only consistently found under certain stressful conditions, mainly under social stress. The data from this social psychological study add another argument to the hypothesis of behavioral inhibition as a coping style, since inhibition in emotion-expressing behavior reduces the probability of an intact social support system, and thereby increases the vulnerability to suffer under so-called stress disorders.

Conclusions

Although this review is not a comprehensive one, it does show that the inhibition of emotional expression is an important factor in the development and maintenance of several psychosomatic disorders. Reduced expressiveness can be viewed as a risk factor (Traue & Kraus, 1988). There are some superficial similarities between the concept of alexithymia and inhibited emotional expression, though the first is a very broad and weak concept based on the observation of reduced cognitive activity with respect to emotional phantasies. In contrast, the concept of inhibited emotional expressiveness is operationalized as a deficit of overt expressiveness, and is based on the psychobiological mechanisms of a behavioral inhibitory system or introversion in the newer conceptualization by Gray (1976). A sensitive or overactivated inhibitory system makes an individual vulnerable for specific socialization factors (Buck, 1984) based on learning mechanisms. Although inhibited emotional expressiveness could be identified as a general factor in psychosomatic disorders, its contribution to specific disorders still has to be identified. Therefore, further social psychophysiological research on these specific psychophysiological disorders is necessary.

For clinical practice and research, some conclusions regarding diagnosis, therapy and prevention of psychosomatic disorders and myogenic pain processes can be drawn:

1. *Diagnosis.* Reduced nonverbal expressiveness or, more generally, behavioral inhibition is not necessarily a personality dimension that is independent of situational factors. As the experimental studies showed, it occurs more probably under certain stressful encounters, particularly in social stress situations, which are to be classified in the group of so-called natural stress conditions. Therefore, the assessment of nonverbal expressiveness should be made in standardized stressful social situations. They can be selected from the videotaped behavioral analytic interview or from a role-play situation. Subjective instruments like the *Affective Communication Test* (Friedman, Prince, Riggio, & Dimatteo, 1985) can only support the diagnosis and result in additional informations. The videotaped behavioral data have to be coded and rated by using a system of behavioral scales which allow interindividual comparisions and the comparison with normative data. However, this implicates the need for normative behavior data of emotional expressiveness. Otherwise information about emotional behavior will stay in the realm of non-reliable clinical observations or on the other hand as research methods without any clinical relevance.

2. *Therapy.* Different psychotherapeutic interventions include strategies to improve emotional expressive behavior. Some psychodynamic therapeutic studies show the effectiveness of expressiveness training. However, only recently have specific clinical procedures to improve overt emotional responding in social stressful situations been developed. An example is a therapeutic program with behaviorally oriented strategies to train expressiveness, the interaction with other persons and the perception of internal emotional impulses (Gerber, 1982). This therapy proved to be very efficient in the treatment of pain patients. In addition to biofeedback Hudzinski (1984) trained headache patients to activate their facial muscles in order to improve their discrimination abilities. Although not conceptualizing it as expressiveness training, he instructed his patients to produce emotional facial signs. Therefore, the therapeutic effects might be—at least in parts—due to the improvement of emotion expression abilities.

Independent of the theoretical background of a therapeutic strategy or setting, there might be a general effect with respect to the self-disclosure by the patient. High self-disclosers, however, improve their cognitive complexity since new points of view (from the therapist) are introduced to the individual's thinking, and consequently the social support improves (Pennebaker, 1985). It remains the problem of a differential indication which depends on diagnostic procedures, and the development of more sophisticated and specific behavioral procedures to reduce behavioral inhibition and improve emotional expressiveness.

3. *Prevention.* Recent studies with children show that there might be a genetic factor influencing the individual differences of expressive behavior. Field, Woodson, Greenberg, and Cohen (1982) demonstrated in neonates an inverse relationship between expressiveness and being irritated when undergoing a neurological examination. In addition, several studies show the importance of socialization conditions (Buck, 1984). Put together, these data speak for a sensitivity of nonexpressive children to become bodily aroused under stress and even more nonexpressive as a consequence of constitutional and learning factors. This obviously constitutes a risk factor. Therefore, attention has to be paid to parental upbringing behavior. Particularly dangerous are those child-rearing styles that include punishment of overt emotional expressiveness. Unfortunately, this style of parental upbringing is quite common in Western societies—as is a high incidence of clinically relevant pain in school children (Zenz, Balzer-Böken, Terpeluk, Traue, & Wehner, 1985).

References

Anderson, C.D. (1981). Expression of affect and physiological response in psychosomatic patients. *Journal of Psychosomatic Research, 25,* 143.

Bischoff, C., & Traue H.C. (1983). Myogenic headache. In K.A. Holroyd, B. Schlote & H. Zenz (Eds.), *Perspectives in research on headache* (pp. 66—90). Toronto/Lewiston, NY: C.J. Hogrefe.

Brady, J.V. (1975). Toward a behavioral biology of emotion. In L. Levi (Ed.), *Emotion: Their parameters and measurement.* New York: Raven Press.

Brooks, G.R., & Richardson, F.C. (1980). Emotional skills training: A treatment program for duodenal ulcer. *Behavior Therapy, 11,* 198—207.

Buck, R. (1979). Individual differences in nonverbal sending accuracy and electrodermal responding: The externalizing-internalizing dimension. In R. Rosenthal (Ed.), *Skills in nonverbal communication.* Cambridge, MA: Oelgeschlager, Gunn & Hain.

Buck, R. (1984). *The communication of emotion.* New York/London: Guilford.

Byrne, D. (1961). The repression-sensitization scale. Rationale, reliability and validity. *Journal of Personality, 29,* 334—349.

Cobb, S. (1976). Social support as a moderation of life stress. *Psychosomatic Medicine, 38,* 300—314.

Engel, B.T. (1986). Psychosomatic medicine, behavioral medicine, just plain medicine. *Psychosomatic Medicine, 48,* 466—479.

Field, T.M., Woodson, R., Greenberg, R., & Cohen, D. (1982). Discrimination and imitation of facial expressions in neonates. *Science, 218,* 179—181.

Flor, H., Turk, D.C., & Birbaumer, N. (1985). Assessment of stress-related psychophysiological reactions in chronic back pain patients. *Journal of Consulting and Clinical Psychology, 53,* 354—364.

Florin, I. (1985). Bewältigungsverhalten und Krankheit. In H.-D. Basler & I. Florin (Eds.), *Klinische Psychologie und körperliche Krankheit.* Stuttgart: Kohlhammer.

Florin, I., Freudenberg, G., & Hollaender, J. (1985). Facial expressions of emotion and physiological reactions in children with bronchial asthma. *Psychosomatic Medicine, 47*(3), 382—393.

Friedman, H.S., Prince, L.M., Riggio, R.E., & Dimatteo, M.R. (1985). Understanding and assessing nonverbal expressiveness: The affective communication test. *Journal of Personality and Social Psychology, 39,* 333—351.
Gambaro, A., & Rabin, S. (1969). Diastolic blood pressure response following direct and displaced aggression after anger arousal, in high and low guilt subjects. *Journal of Personality and Social Psychology, 12,* 87—94.
Gannon, L. R. (1981). The psychophysiology of psychosomatic disorders. In S.N. Haynes & L. Gannon (Eds.), *Psychosomatic disorders.* New York: Praeger.
Gerber, W.D. (1982). Uni- und multidimensionale Therapieansätze. In W.D. Gerber & G. Haag (Eds.), *Migräne.* Berlin/Heidelberg/New York: Springer-Verlag.
Gray, J.A. (1976). The behavioral inhibition system: A possible substrate for anxiety. In M.P. Feldman & A.M. Broodhurst (Eds.), *Theoretical and experimental base of behavior modification.* New York: Wiley.
Hokanson, J.E., & Burgess, M. (1962). The effects of three types of aggression on vascular processes. *Journal of Abnormal and Social Psychology, 64,* 446—449.
Hollaender, J., & Florin, I. (1983). Expressed emotion and airway conductance in children with bronchial asthma. *Journal of Psychosomatic Research, 27*(4), 307—311.
Hudzinski, L.G. (1984). The significance of muscle discrimination training in the treatment of chronic muscle contraction headache. *Headache, 24,* 203—210.
Jäger, R., Lischer, S., Münster, B., & Ritz, B. (1976). *Biographisches Inventar zur Diagnose von Verhaltensstörungen (BIV).* Göttingen: Hogrefe.
Jones, H.E. (1935). The galvanic skin response as related to overt emotional expression. *American Journal of Psychology, 47,* 241—257.
Katz, F., Wittkower, E.D., Vavruska, G.W., Telner, P., & Ferguson, S. (1957). Studies on vascular skin responses in atopic dermatitis: The influence of psychological factors. *Journal of Investigative Dermatology, 29,* 67—78.
Lazarus, R.S. (1966). *Psychological stress and the coping process.* New York: McGraw-Hill.
Malatesta, C.Z., Jonas, R., & Izard, C.E. (1987). The relation between low facial expressivity during emotional arousal and somatic symptoms. *British Journal of Medical Psychology, 60,* 169—180.
Meissner, S.J. (1977). Family process in psychosomatic disease. In Z.J. Lipowski, R.D. Lipsitt & P.D. Whybrow (Eds.), *Psychosomatic medicine.* New York: University Press.
Pennebaker, J.W. (1985). Traumatic experience and psychosomatic disease: Exploring the roles of behavioral inhibition, obsession and confiding. *Canadian Psychology, 26*(2), 82—94.
Pennebaker, J.W., & Hoover, C.W. (1986) Inhibition and Cognition: Toward an understanding of trauma and disease. In R.J. Davidson, G.F. Schwartz, & D. Shapiro (Eds.), *Consciousness and self-regulation, Vol. 4.* New York: Plenum.
Ruesch, S. (1948). The infantile personality — the core problem of psychosomatic medicine. *Psychosomatic Medicine, 10,* 134—144.
Schlote, B.M. (1987). *Psychophysiologische Verlaufsuntersuchung von SKS: Eine Feldstudie.* Ulm: PSZ-Verlag.
Schwartz, G.E. (1983). Social psychophysiology and behavioral medicine: A systems perspective. In J.T. Cacioppo, R.E. Petty & D. Shapiro (Eds.), *Social psychophysiology.* New York: Guilford.
Seitz, P.F.D. (1953). Dynamically oriented brief psychotherapy: Psychocoutanous exoriation syndroms, an experiment. *Psychosomatic Medicine, 15,* 200.
Sifneos, P.E. (1973). The prevalence of alexithymic characteristics in psychosomatic patients. *Psychotherapy and Psychosomatics, 22,* 255—262.

Sternbach, R.A. (1966). *Principles of psychophysiology* (1971, 3rd ed.). New York/London: Academic Press.
Stokvis, B. (1953). Het probleem van de "specificiteit" in de psychosomatische geneeskunde, structur analytisch benadert. *Ned. T. Geneesh., 97,* 3043—3050.
Traue, H.C. (in press). *Gefühlsausdruck. Hemmung und Muskelspannung.* Göttingen: Hogrefe.
Traue, H.C., Bischoff, C., & Zenz, H. (1986). Sozialer Streß, Muskelspannung und Spannungskopfschmerz. *Zeitschrift für Klinische Psychologie, 15,* 57—70.
Traue, H.C., Gottwald, A., Henderson, P.R., & Bakal, D.A. (1985). Nonverbal expressiveness and EMG activity in tension headache sufferers and controls. *Journal of Psychosomatic Research, 29,* 375—381.
Traue, H.C., & Knaus, S. (submitted). Nonverbale Expressivität und soziale Unterstützung bei chronischen Kopfschmerzen. *Zeitschrift für Klinische Psychologie.*
Traue, H.C., & Kraus, W. (1988). Ausdruckshemmung als Risikofaktor: Eine verhaltensmedizinische Analyse. *Praxis der klinischen Verhaltensmedizin und Rehabilitation, 2,* 89—95.
Tunis, M.M., & Wolff, H.G. (1954). Studies on headache: Cranial artery vasoconstriction and muscle contraction headache. *Archives of Neurology and Psychiatry, 71,* 425—434.
Weiner, H. (1977). *Psychobiology and human disease.* New York/Oxford/Amsterdam: Elsevier.
Wittkower, E.D., & Lipowski, Z.J. (1966). Recent developments in psychosomatic medicine. *Psychosomatic Medicine, 28,* 722—737.
Wolff, H.G. (1937). Personality features and reactions of subjects with migraine. *Archives of Neurology and Psychiatry, 37,* 895—921.
Zenz, H, Balzer-Böken, B., Terpeluk, V., Traue, H.C., & Wehner, C. (1985). *Unterschiede im Körperbeschwerdebild von Schülern vor, während und nach der Pubertät.* Unpublished research report, University of Ulm.

Long-Term Registration of Muscle Tension among Office Workers Suffering from Tension Headache

Barbara Schlote

The results of studies on muscle tension in tension headache sufferers have been contradictory possibly because experimental conditions lacked ecological validity. The present study investigates whether tension headache sufferers exhibit increased levels of muscle tension in ecologically valid situations.

A field study was carried out in a large area office of an insurance company. Fifteen full-time employees particitaped: 9 subjects suffered from tension headache symptoms, 6 were painfree controls. The trapezius EMG was registered for almost 7 hours during 5 working-days. All the participants kept a headache diary and reported the amount of stress at work.

Average levels in the trapezius EMG were significantly increased in headache sufferes compared to painfree controls. There was no difference in the EMG levels of headache sufferers when periods of time with and without pain were compared. Individuals with tension headache reported significantly less stress than painfree controls.

Results support the hypothesis of increased muscle effort in tension headache sufferers proposed by Bischoff and Traue (1983). The lack of increased EMG levels during pain episodes may be due to the low intensity of pain. The possibility of perceptual deficits is discussed with respect to low stress reports and elevated levels of muscle tension in tension headache sufferers.

Lately, there have been increasing doubts as to whether tension headaches should be considered a separate class of headaches. The reason for this lies in the contradictory results of numerous psychophysiological experiments conducted to demonstrate the existence of a type of headache caused by muscle tension.

Classifying a form of headache as muscle contraction headache (the term tension headache is often used synonymously) goes back to the Ad Hoc Committee for the classification of headaches (Friedman et al., 1962). The definition of this class of headaches contains a number of vague statements concerning the physiological concomitants and the etiology of this type of headache.

The vagueness of these statements led to the deduction of assumptions. Philips (1978) has made a trenchant list of these. In over 20 years of investigation into headaches, researchers have tried to find psychophysiological group differences, yielding etiological clues, between persons with tension headaches, those with migraine, and subjects free of any pain. A review and discussion of

---

Translated by Jennifer Hartog.

experiments concerning some of the most frequently tested assumptions has been published by Schlote (1987).

Altogether, the results can hardly make a strong case for the assumption that tension headache sufferers differ from subjects with migraine or persons not suffering from headache in the tension of their head and neck muscles. I think it is a remarkable fact that hardly any of these studies give any clues explaining the basis of their assumption.

If we are to compare the results of the tests done on each particular muscle, it becomes apparent—and especially striking as far as the EMG in a situation of relief is concerned—that the number of differences found between groups is relatively small compared with the total number of tests done for one particular muscle. It is further striking how low the EMG values, measured in stress situations, usually are. The stress conditions were so seldom felt to be stressful that sometimes even the main effect for the stress was missing. The main reason was probably the limited "ecological validity" of the stress conditions (for too short a period, bringing about stress under physically relaxing conditions).

A further methodological problem is that the definition of tension headaches given by the Ad Hoc Committee hardly gives reliable criteria for diagnosing a headache as belonging to the group of tension headaches. The criteria used in the experiments for selecting subjects with tension headaches vary. A selection of tension headache sufferers chosen according to positive criteria of tension headaches is rare. In short, the design of the experiments was seldom suited to test whether such a form of headache exists which is accompanied by increased muscle activity and/or which could be a result of it.

In order to answer this question, the same subjects should have their EMG measured between, before, and during episodes of tension headaches. This approach was followed in case studies in the early phase of psychophysiological headache research—often, however, without their being part of the headache diagnosis. Tunis and Wolff (1954) and Simons et al. (1943) discovered an increase of the EMG during the headache episodes. More recent studies, which compared different groups of subjects, found elevated values in the frontalis EMG during the pain phase just as much among subjects with tension headaches (Haynes et al., 1975) as among subjects suffering from migraine (Bakal & Kaganov, 1977). During the attack, the migraineurs also had an increased trapezius EMG. Three other studies (Martin & Mathews, 1978; Philips 1977, 1978) could not find any increase in the EMG during the headache phases. These experiments were also conducted in laboratories so that the points made above concerning such experiments apply (more or less) here, too. The experimental setting does not allow much behavioral elbow-room.

Following Bischoff and Traue's (1983) model of myogenic headache we can, however, assume that persons suffering from headaches differ from persons not prone to headaches in the very way in which they typically react to situations. Bischoff and Traue developed a model to explain the origin of myogenic headaches in which they hypothesize that subjects develop a headache—in the sense of myogenic headache—when muscle activity increases above a critical point within a certain period of time in situations of stress or relief (the "hypothesis of increased muscle activity"). Bischoff and Sauermann (in this volume) assume that deficits in the perception both of stressing situations and of muscle tension play a determining role in the origin of increased muscle activity.

Bischoff and Traue (1983) distinguish five possibilities of how dysfunctional muscle tension, i.e., inadequate reactions to the situation, can appear. Compared to pain-free subjects, muscle tension among persons with tension headache (1) increases in stressful situations and (2) decreases more slowly after a stressful situation, whereas (3) subjects prone to tension headaches have an increased level of muscle tension even in a situation of relief. Some tension headache sufferers do show functional muscle reactions in some situations of stress; it is (4) the accumulation of stressful situations they have to cope with which is dysfunctional, as is the amount of increased muscle tension which it involves. In the same way, some persons tend to stay longer in a stressful situation, which means that they have (5) increased muscle tension for a longer period of time. On the basis of the ideas put forth above, I examine in this paper the pattern of muscle tension among individuals presenting clear symptoms of tension headache, studied under natural and individually relevant stress conditions.

Ideas on the possible pathophysiology of myogenic pain have helped determine the site where muscle tension should be measured. Bischoff and Traue (1983) showed how muscle activity can lead to pain in the form of tension headaches. Static contraction activity of over 15% of maximal muscle tension, lasting for an extended period of time, can cause an ischemic state: the blood pH-level drops, which, in turn, leads to the release of chemical pain substances (such as bradykinin, serotonin, and prostaglandin), bringing down the threshold for mechano-sensitive nociceptors. Persisting pain may develop when the pain itself causes a reflex increase of muscle tension; central influences such as emotional factors (fear, anger), which often appear in stress situations, play a decisive role in the generation of reflex contractions.

The location of pain caused by tension does not necessarily have to be the same as the place where tension occurs. Travell (1976; Travell & Rinzler, 1952) demonstrated that the stimulation of certain points in various muscles caused pain in certain other zones. The anatomical and physiochemical nature of the trigger-points and the physiological mechanism of the transmitted pain has remained almost totally unexplained to date. Muscles that might be considered for the location of pain typical for the pain in tension headaches are:

- m.sternocleidomastoideus with pain projection to the lateral frontal area (amongst other places),
- m. splenius capitis with pain projection zones in the vertex and surrounding area,
- m. temporalis with pain projection toward the eyebrows and other areas,

— m. trapezius, pars descendens with pain projection from the neck to the occipital area and the parietal to the temporal area.

According to the experience of the Department of Medical Psychology of the University of Ulm, the pain pattern of many patients with the symptoms of tension headache corresponds to an origin of pain in the upper m. trapezius area: Pain starts in the neck and proceeds, often bilaterally, toward the frontal area. Furthermore, in experiments using relatively "real" social stressors, especially the m. trapezius showed the differences between subjects with tension headaches and a control group (Traue, Bischoff, & Zenz, 1981; Traue et al., 1985). Thus, it seemed sensible to register the EMG of the trapezius in order to test the hypothesis that tension headache symptoms are linked to elevated levels of muscle tension.

The aim of this study was to find clues for the myogenity of tension headache symptoms by registring the trapezius EMG over a longer period of time; it was important to follow the subjects in stressful situations with higher ecological validity. This approach allows the observation of muscular dysfunctions—that is, if they exist at all. Since Howarth (1965) and Dhopesh et al. (1980) noticed that stress at work is one of the factors triggering headaches other than migraine, and since portable instruments for EMG registration have since been developed and used profitably for field studies (Marschall, 1983; Rugh, 1979; Rugh & Solberg, 1976), we decided to measure the EMG over a longer period of time in a normal work setting.

We expected the following results:

— *Hypothesis 1:* Tension headache sufferers would produce more muscle activity during a working day than would pain-free individuals with comparable work.
— *Hypothesis 2:* During breaks, tension headache sufferers would also be more tense.
— *Hypothesis 3:* Muscle tension would increase just before the onset of the headache.
— *Hypothesis 4:* During a headache attack, muscle tension would be higher than during headache-free periods.
— *Hypothesis 5:* With reference to Bischoff and Sauermann's research (in this volume), we assumed that tension headache sufferers would not be able to include increases of muscular tension in their judgement of strain owing to perceptual deficits, i.e., their stress ratings would be lower.
— *Hypothesis 6:* The pain itself and the fear of pain increase represent a considerable additional stress factor for headache sufferers (Bakal, 1982). Hence our hypothesis that the work load is considered to be more taxing during headache periods than during pain-free intervals.

Method

The study took place in the open-plan office of the local health insurance (Allgemeine Ortskrankenkasse, AOK) in Ulm. The conditions at work were almost the same for all the employees: identical furniture, air-conditioning, similar sound level, wall-to-wall carpeting treated against static electricity).

Selection of the Subjects

A short questionnaire concerning headaches worked out by the Department of Medical Psychology was sent to all of the 160 full-time employees of the AOK. The subjects were chosen among the employees who wrote that they "never" or "hardly ever" had a headache and those who "almost always," "several times a week," or "several times a month" suffered from headaches which started slowly with a feeling of tension or pain in the neck or at the back of the head. A personal interview and a second, more detailed questionnaire relating to these headaches made sure that the subjects in the tension headache group did really present the symptoms of tension headaches: pain starting slowly, sometimes or usually dull and/or constant; occurrence: several times a week; duration: hours or days; localization: often bilateral suboccipital to frontal and hard to localize (Schlote, 1987; Wolf-Cramer 1984). Excluded from the study were those employees who knew their spine to be damaged, who were over 10% overweight (risk of insufficient EMG signals) or whose headaches were due to meningitis or to an accident.

Registration of Muscle Tension

The m. trapezius, pars descendens, was selected for a long-term EMG. We expected subjects prone to headaches to strain this muscle excessively statically while writing. Further, the activity of this muscle could be measured unobtrusively. We used Lippold's standard guidelines (1967), modified by Zipp (1982) to measure the trapezius EMG. We measured on the right-hand side to avoid the disturbing influence from the beating heart. Ag/AgCl electrodes, 10 mm in diameter, made by Hellige were used. The skin of the subjects was prepared so that the coupling resistance of the skin was no more than 5 kΩ (this was checked with the LCD Digital Multitester, model AK 508). The EMG was recorded with a six-channel portable instrument (Zak, Simbach). The preamplification took place outside the instrument in an EMG module (noise level < 0.4 µV, high-pass filter, 50 Hz integrated notch filter and band-pass filter in the range of 100—600 Hz, amplifier and rectifier).

The module was applied securely to the breast or to the abdomen. The signal output was proportional to the EMG signal. It was registered 16 times per minutes, i.e., every 3.75 sec. The mean value was calculated for periods of one minute and stored for further calculations in the 60 kB CMOS-RAM memory of the pocket computer, which was fed by a NiCa accumulator bloc carried around the waist in a 100 × 25 × 165 mm, 525 g bag. The EMG values stored every minute could be related to exact times with help of a built-in quarz clock.

Stress Rating

Since different stress situations can lead to similar physiological reactions, it seemed justified to do a general stress rating and not one specific to certain situations. The subjects were to make a note of what they were doing at what time, and to report on an 11-point scale (from 0 to 10) how much stress they were feeling. At the end of the day, each subject reported on a 100 mm visual analogue scale how stressed he or she had felt, on the whole, during the day.

Recording the Headaches

Each subject recorded his or her headache symptoms at 9 a.m., 11 a.m., 1 p.m., and 3 p.m.. More frequent recordings would probably have disturbed the work schedule as the subjects had to give detailed information. The location of the headaches had to be indicated on two sketched head profiles (left and right), which were divided into several parts according to the location of the muscles (Bakal, 1982). The headache intensity was to be recorded on a 100 mm visual analogue scale. These visual scales correlated highly with the otherwise more usual verbal pain intensity scales (Ohnhaus & Adler, 1975). The quality of pain was to be described with the help of six categories (constant, pulling, pressing, stinging, shooting, and throbbing) and one open category. The subjects were asked each time they recorded the way they felt to say whether any of the 13 possible accompanying symptoms of various forms of headaches applied (e.g., paleness, sweating, chilliness, nausea, photophobia, etc.). Fourteen items were then checked which concerned behavior capable of changing the course of the headache. A separate recording of feelings of tension seemed intuitively to be useful; location and intensity were recorded at the same times and in the same way as the recordings of the headaches.

Recording of Variables which Could Possibly Intervene

Since increases of muscular tension—in the sense of secondary tension—can be caused not only by headaches but also by other ailments, all subjects were asked to list mornings and evenings all complaints that had come up during the experiment. For this purpose we used an abridged and slightly modified version of the *Gießen Symptom Assessment* (GBB, Brähler, 1978). It contained items concerning the areas of exhaustion, stomach ailments, pains in the limbs, heart complaints as well as—and this was new—colds and an open category called "other complaints."

Patients suffering from headaches often mention sleep disorders if the headaches are related to depression (Barolin, 1976). Therefore, individuals had to record the subjective quality of their sleep, the number of times they woke up, and the presumed amount of sleep. The mood of the subjects was recorded with a visual analogue scale before starting work and at the end of the working day. Luria (1975) showed that visual analogue scales are appropriate for such purposes.

Course of the Field Study

We recorded the data on five successive working days from 8 a.m. to 5 p.m. In the morning, the subjects indicated how they had slept the previous night, how they felt, and whether they had any physical complaints. The electrodes were applied for the registration of the trapezius EMG (heart rate and head movements; Schlote, 1987). The instruments and electrodes were checked to make sure they worked. The electrodes, wire, and the EMG module were attached with tape so as not to slide; we made sure that the subjects freedom of movement was not impaired. These preparations lasted about 20 minutes and always took place in the AOK staff medical care rooms.

During the daytime the employees went about their usual activities such as working on files and handing them on to the next department, phoning, talking with insurees, and taking part in meetings. Almost all the employees had about the same lunch break during which each person went about doing the things they usually did at lunch time: shopping, eating in the canteen, or going for a short drive. The afternoons were much like the mornings. In the course of the day, all the subjects had to keep their "headache diary" at the same times.

At the end of their working day, between 3 and 5 p.m., the subjects went one by one to the medical care room. There, they filled out once again the *Gießen Sympton Assessment*, assessed their mood and the day's total stress. A few weeks after the end of the experiment, each subject received DM 150 for their participation.

Treatment of the Raw Data

In order to minimize the number of missing data, we used only the values measured between 8.41 a.m. and 3.20 p.m. which means that we had 400 1-minute muscle tension mean values. These raw data were first stored on a floppy disk (ZAK computer) then transferred for further calculations onto magnetic tapes of a Siemens 7550 computer. The time intervals of stress ratings, related to specific work periods, were weighted with the stress rating (0 to 100); then hourly means were calculated. For our calculations we used the BMDP statistical software package (Dixon et al., 1983) on the TR440, the Siemens 7550 (BS 2000).

Results

Group Comparisons

Muscle tension: We first used a 2-factorial analysis of variance to see whether we could include the measures collected the first day in the analysis of our data, and to see whether there were different reactions according to groups as far as carrying the instruments was concerned. As there was no main effect for the first day of registration, and as the interrelation between group and day of measuring was too slight to create a trend, we included the data collected the first day in our analysis ($p = .11$).

In order to test the first hypothesis that employees with tension headaches had more total muscle tension than pain-free employees, we calculated the arithmetical mean of the subjects for all the days of our study. We tested the homogeneity of variance using the Levene test and found a standard distribution of the muscle tension means in both groups. The t-test for homogeneous samples confirmed the hypothesis that, on the whole, employees suffering from headaches have increased muscle effort compared with employees without any pain complaints (group of headache sufferers: 27.1 µV, control group: 17.1 µV; $p = .05$).

Figure 1 shows the EMG values of the average day. We calculated the "hourly" means for each group for the following time spans: 8.41—9.30 a.m., 9.31—10.30 a.m ... 1.31—2.30 p.m., 2.31—3.20 p.m. At all times the group of headache sufferers had increased muscle effort compared with the control group.

Employees suffering from tension headache symptoms had significantly higher levels of muscle tension values than the control subjects not only during the lunch break (12.31 p.m.—1.30 p.m.) but also during the working hours in the morning and in the afternoon (total: $p < 0.5$) (hypothesis 2) (Table 1).

Stress Ratings

We checked the fifth hypothesis that employees with tension headaches rate the extent of their daily stress as being less than employees without any pain problems by group comparisons of stress assessments of specific activities and of the retrospective assessment of the whole day. Mann-Whitney's U-test (Claus & Ebner, 1971) revealed that employees suffering from headaches wrote down significantly lower values—for both stress ratings—than the employees in the control group (Table 2).

The average daily pattern of the stress ratings in both groups was that of an upside down U-curve in the morning followed by a new increase in the afternoon after the drop during the lunch break (Schlote, 1987). At all times, but especially from 10.31 a.m. to 2.30 p.m., did the headache sufferers feel they were less under

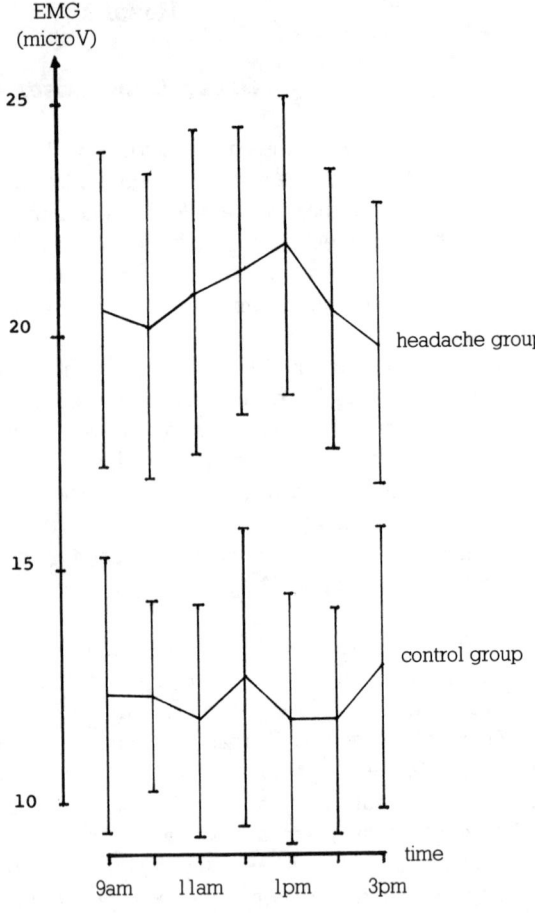

Figure 1. Average trapezius EMG through a day for employees with and without headache problems.

Table 1. Comparison of the trapezius-EMG (micro V): employees suffering from headaches and pain-free employes.

	headache sufferers	control group	p <
whole day	27.1	17.1	.05
morning	26.1	17.3	.05
lunchtime	27.9	16.3	.05
afternoon	25.6	17.5	.05

Table 2. Comparison of stress ratings of employees with headaches and that of pain-free employees: retrospective rating of the whole day and activity-related stress rating (range of values: 0–100).

	employees with headaches	employees without headaches	p <
retrospective stress rating	36.0	59.7	.01
activity related stress rating	37.9	52.9	.05

stress than did the control subjects. There was no interaction between group and time of rating. Both groups felt much less stressed during the lunch break.

The average correlation between stress and muscle tension was .023 for the headache sufferers and .175 for the pain-free subjects. In certain cases, there were also significant positive correlations between stress ratings and muscle tension values.

Sleep, mood and feeling of physical well-being: Our analysis of the daily reports showed that there were no differences between the groups with respect to quality of sleep, length of sleep, number of sleep interruptions during the night, and mood. All the differences were tested for significance with Mann-Whitney's U-test (Claus & Ebner, 1971). The only significant difference was the estimated time span between waking up in the morning and actually getting up: 30 minutes for the subjects suffering from headaches and 11 minutes for the pain-free subjects ($p = .02$).

There were no differences between the groups either concerning exhaustion, stomach ailments, heart trouble, or other complaints (Mann-Whitney's U-test). As expected, the headache sufferers reported significantly more pains in the limbs ($p = .02$) than did the pain-free subjects. This is because some of the items on that scale were related to headaches. Altogether, we can state that the control subjects had hardly any complaints, and that the headache sufferers only had headaches and the symptoms which go along with them.

Description of Headaches

During the time we were collecting the data, all the employees in the headache group developed a headache or feelings of tension at least once. As far as headaches were concerned, we had complete data for 19 out of 20 possible moments (4 entries and 5 days); data on tension ratings were collected 18.9 times on average. Altogether, headaches were mentioned 76 times and feelings of tension 87 times; in 43 cases the headache was accompanied by feelings of tension. On average, 44% of the time (8.4 out of 19 entries) the headache sufferers had headaches and 51% of the time (9.6 out of 18.9) they felt tense.

Location of the complaints: The most common complaints were feelings of tension in the neck (76% the right part of the neck, and 48% the left part of the neck). The shoulders were often tense, too. In comparison, other locations were seldom tense.

Pain was mostly felt in the forehead: on the left side on average 4 times and on the right side 3.7 times per headache sufferer, i.e., 47% and 43% of all the headache entries. The subjects complained every now and then of pains at the back of the head and the top of the head.

The pain was described as "pressure" (35 times), as "constant" (33 times), "dull" (22 times), "stinging" (13 times), or "pulling" pain (7 times); "throbbing" "shooting," and the other qualifiers were not mentioned at all. The accompanying symptoms were mostly stiffness in the neck (46%). Symptoms concerning the eyes were mentioned relatively often too: pressure on eyes (33%), photophobia (22%), runny eyes (18%); a band-like pressure around the head was mentioned in only 13% of the cases.

Comparison of the Periods With and Without Headaches

On average, both the absolute number of entries concerning headaches and feelings of tension and the figures for headaches and tension weighted with their intensity were equally distributed across the 4 times of daily registration (Figure 2). Feelings of tension among the headache sufferers increased noticeably, yet not significantly, between 9 a.m. and 11 a.m. The slight increase of the intensity of headaches toward the afternoon was of no statistical importance either. The intensity of the headaches was generally relatively low: on average 25 on the 100 mm visual analogue scale (maximum 54). Headache intensities of less than 10 were not considered for data analysis.

Hypothesis 4 stated that muscle tension would be increased during the headache periods. In contrast to this hypothesis, we found out that the average EMG for the headache-free periods was identical to that of the headache periods: 27.2 µV in each case (average headache intensity: 25).

Muscle tension: We were not able to test the third hypothesis as to whether muscle tension is increased just before the onset of a headache, or whether it increases even more during the headache episode, since there were not enough cases with all the data. For seven headache episodes (two from a single subject), we had data covering the hour before onset, the first hour during onset of the headache, and an equivalent—as far as time is concerned—hour without any headache. We found no indications for a usual EMG increase before or during the onset of headaches.

Using the Wilcoxon test, we tested the difference in average individual stress ratings between periods with and without headaches (hypothesis 6). As a result, stress evaluations during headache episodes equaled those during pain-free intervals: 44 arbitrary units (visual analogue scale). Visual inspection of data on in-

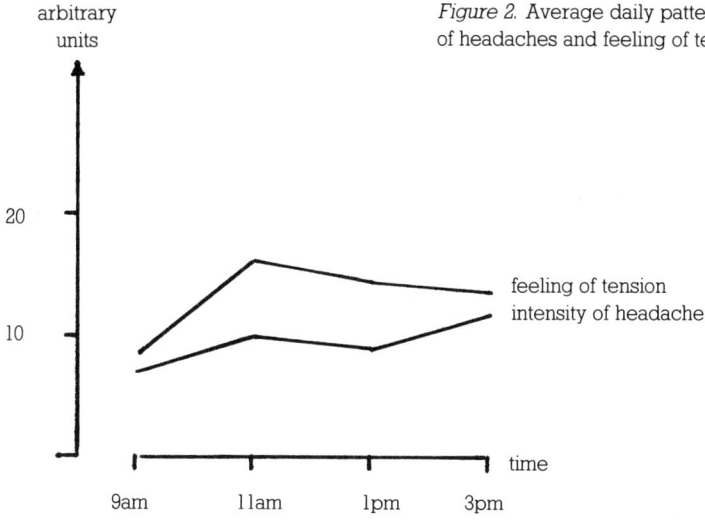

Figure 2. Average daily pattern of intensity of headaches and feeling of tension.

tensity ratings, stress-ratings, and EMG averages revealed no relationship between these variables.

Interpretation

As its main result, this study was able to demonstrate that employees suffering from tension headache symptoms need much more muscle effort than employees without pain problems when doing comparable normal desk work. The difference between groups continued throughout the entire time at work and during lunch break as well. Average daily EMG scores varied between 25.9 µV and 27.9 µV in employees with tension headaches and between 15.4 µV and 18.8 µV in pain-free controls, respectively. There was one exception: One female headache sufferer achieved an average of only 7.8 µV and 1-minute maxima of 30 µV. Mistakes in measurement could be excluded. Sweetman et al. (1980) reported a similar and unexplainable phenomenon at the Symposium on Ambulatory Recording in 1980 with respect to EMG registrations in low back pain.

During the course of a working day, EMG scores changed little in either group. This observation matches studies in which the EMG of individuals engaged in full-time work in a sitting position was registered (Lille & Cheliout, 1982).

The result of elevated m. trapezius levels in employees with muscle tension symptoms supports the hypothesis of increased muscle effort put forth by the Ulm headache research group (Bischoff & Traue, 1983; Bischoff et al., 1986). This hypothesis states that individuals with tension headaches exert more muscle effort within a certain period of time than individuals without tension headaches. Inferences about the "critical amount" of increased muscle effort are, however, premature. Average scores of muscle tension in the tension headache group as well as in the control group clearly exceeded those registered in the same muscle in stress experiments (with similar registration techniques: Traue, Bischoff, & Zenz, 1981; Bischoff, Traue, & Zenz, 1982). The majority of stress experiments with tension headache sufferers did not produce significant results (Schlote, 1987). In most of these experiments, situations were highly structured and lacking behavioral elbow-room (remain seated, often in a reclining chair, relaxation instruction before/after exposure to stressor, etc.). Naturally occurring stressful situations often lacked fixed structures and time limits. There are reasons to believe that in these types of situations, tension headache sufferers tend to choose dysfunctional, e.g., static postures that promote muscle tension (Traue et al., 1985). This interpretation is supported by the fact that the employees were able to relax their m.trapezius just as much as employees without pain problems were. Every working day, many 1-minute averages of the trapezius EMG were well below those registered by Bischoff, Traue, and Zenz (1982) or Traue et al. (1985) when they instructed students with and without tension headache problems to relax (Jacobson). Except for one pain-free employee and one with headaches, all the employees had at least one 1-minute score of less than 5 µV every day; many individuals had 1-minute averages of less than 3 µV.

Since clerical work puts particular strain on the m. trapezius, it would be functional to relax this muscle during breaks. Yet muscle tension in the control group decreased only minimally during lunch breaks, while EMG scores in the tension headache group slightly increased (but not significantly), despite the elevation of scores during work.

Stress Rating

Employees with tension headaches gave a lower rating to their feelings of stress than the controls did. This was the case for activity-related as well as for retrospective evaluations of the whole working day despite increased muscle tension in this group. Group differences came out more clearly in retrospective evaluations. Average scores for the 5-day registration period ran from between 17 and 49 arbitrary units on the visual analogue scale for headache sufferers (except for one with 58), and from between 44 and 77 units in pain-free controls.

Work-related evaluations of stress ranged between 25 and 59 in the headache group and between 44 and 69 in the control group (one individual averaged 29). Group differences in work-related stress ratings arose mainly from differences in stress evaluations in the morning and during the lunch break. There were no sex differences.

If we take Bischoff's (1989) reflections into account on the development of assessments of effort regarding activities with moderate static strain, we should expect that signals from the m.trapezius, a muscle that is particularly involved in clerical work, would modify the assessment of subjective stress. This does not seem to be the case, however. Average correlations between the evaluation of stress and muscle tension almost equal zero in either group. The general tendency of the headache group to feel only little stress, on the one hand, and to exhibit elevated levels of muscle tension on the other, could point to a perceptual deficit in tension headache sufferers. Experiments by Bischoff (1989) revealed that individuals with tension headaches are less able to perceive proprioceptive signals, so that they underestimate the total amount of effort.

Complaints

This field study succeeded in finding a group among the 160 employees of the AOK, which, although small, contained individuals who clearly suffered from symptoms of tension headache but from no other physical complaints. The employees who served as controls were completely free from physical complaints.

Each employee of the headache group had a headache at least once during the time of registration. Most of the headaches reached only moderate intensity; they never led to vomiting. Following the "continuum model" proposed by Bakal (1980, 1982), the headaches should be classified at one end of the continuum as the mild nonproblematic form of the muscle tension type. In contrast to the model, headaches reported in this study were accompanied by visual symptoms of vascular origin among musculoskeletal and autonomous symptoms. Since development and quality of pain were more characteristic of tension headache than of migraine, these headaches can be considered to be a mixed form.

Headaches were frequently located in the frontal or orbital area with the left side being more often involved than the right side. Pain in the occipital region and neck occurred more often on the right side (one-quarter of all pain episodes) than on the left side (one-fifth of all episodes). The surplus of complaints in the right part of the neck and occipital region is probably due to clerical activities, which were mainly carried out with the right hand. Frequency and combinations of pain and feelings of tension varied between employees but without any apparent regularity. During registration periods, the intensity of pain tended to be low; there was no diurnal rhythm in intensity ratings. Some subjects, however, reported considerable increases in pain intensity in the evening. Studies on the diurnal variation of pain perception were able to show an increase in the course of the day (Davis et al., 1978) or found reduced pain perception in the morning (Pöllmann & Hildebrandt, 1979; Procacci, 1972, in Glynn & Floyd, 1975). Reduced pain perception and reduced sensibility in the morning (ability to discriminate between two stimuli of differing intensity) is probably due to diurnal variation in endorphin precursors (Davis, Buchsbaum, & Bunney, 1978). In addition, Glynn and Floyd (1975) found that individuals with intractable pain syndromes who had a job outside of the home hardly ever reported increases in pain intensity while at work. Worsening of pain began at about 4 p.m.. Work seems to suppress the diurnal rhythm in pain perception. It possibly distracts attention from physical sensations. The effect of factors that suppress the perception of pain are probably the reason for much lower pain ratings during registration periods (x = 25) than those made in the questionnaires used for selection (x = 53.5).

There was hardly any diurnal variation in the ratings of tension, except that group means tended to be lower at 9 a.m. than at 11 a.m.. The increase of feelings of tension in the morning may have been due to a high work load at this time.

Muscle Tension and Stress Ratings During Headache Episodes

Contrary to all expectations, muscle tension increased neither in the hour before onset of headache nor during pain episodes when compared with pain-free intervals. Trapezius EMG averages during pain episodes equaled those registered in pain-free intervals. Visual inspection of variations in pain intensity ratings and EMG averages did not reveal any similarity at all. Many headache attacks were accompanied by feelings of muscle tension, but again there was no similarity in the variation of either. This study confirms results of other studies, which failed to find a correlation between headache intensity and EMG (van Boxtel & Goudswaard, 1984; Pozniak-Patewicz, 1976; Anderson & Franks, 1981; Harper & Steger, 1978; Philips & Hunter, 1982).

According to experiments of the group around Wolff (e.g., Simons et al., 1943) and theoretical considerations by Bakal (1982), we would expect an increase in muscle tension as a reflex to pain. The absence of any muscle tension increase in this study may be due to the low or moderate intensity of pain. Nor does this study confirm Bakal's (1982) hypothesis that the expectation of possible headache attacks and particularly the attack itself would provoke additional feelings of stress in the individual. The amount of stress experienced during headache episodes did not change. We doubt that this is due to the low intensity of the headaches. From experience, some employees expected a worsening of pain in the evening. A dissociation between muscle tension and pain, however, should only develop in the course of a longer headache history when headaches have become more severe (Bakal, 1980; Traue et al., 1985). In this study, headache episodes can hardly be classified as "troublesome" or "severe" in Bakal's sense. The lack of muscle tension increase during headache episodes, or at least the lack of muscle tension increases before the onset of headache episodes, argues against a direct causal relationship between muscle tension and headache. Yet, the hypothesis of increased muscle effort as well as the hypothesis of perceptual deficits do not lose their validity. The existence of perceptual deficits has been clearly confirmed in experiments by Bischoff (1989; Bischoff & Sauermann, this volume). Slight but constantly increased levels of muscle tension in subjects of the headache group seem to be of symptomatic significance.

References

Anderson, C.D., & Franks, R.D. (1981). Migraine and tension headache: Is there a physiological difference? *Headache, 21,* 63—72.
Bakal, D.A. (1980). Headache. In R.H. Woody (Ed.), *Encyclopedia of clinical assessment, Vol. 1* (pp. 308—318). San Francisco-Washington-London: Jossey-Bass.
Bakal, D.A. (1982). *The psychobiology of chronic headache.* New York: Springer Publishing Co.
Bakal, D.A., & Kaganov, J.A. (1977). Muscle contraction and migraine headache. Psychophysiologic comparison. *Headache, 17,* 208—215.
Barolin, G.S. (1976). Über das Zusammenspiel psychischer und somatischer Faktoren beim Kopfschmerz. *Fortschr. Neurol. Psychiat., 44,* 597—614.
Bischoff, C. (1989). *Wahrnehmung von Muskelspannung. Eine signalentdeckungstheoretische Analyse bei Personen mit Muskelkontraktionskopfschmerz.* Göttingen: Hogrefe.
Bischoff, C., & Traue, H.C. (1983). Mygogenic headache. In K.A. Holroyd, B. Schlote & H. Zenz (Eds.), *Perspectives in research on headache* (pp. 66—90). Toronto/Lewiston, NY: C.J. Hogrefe.
Bischoff, C., Traue, H.C. & Zenz, H. (1982). Muskelspannung und Schmerzerleben von Personen mit und ohne Spannungskopfschmerzen bei experimentell gesetzter aversiver Reizung. *Z. exp. angew. Psychol., 29,* 357—385.
Bischoff, C., Zenz, H., & Traue, H.C. (1986). Primärer Kopfschmerz. In R. Adler, J.M. Herrmann, K. Koehle, O. Schonecke, Th. von Uexküll & W. Wesiak (Eds.), *Psychosomatische Medizin* (pp. 565—582). München: Urban & Schwarzenberg.
Van Boxtel, A., & Goudswaard, P. (1984). Absolute and proportional resting EMG levels in chronic headache patients in relation to state of headache. *Headache, 24,* 259—265.
Brähler, E. (1978). *Der Gießener Beschwerdebogen (GBB).* Habilitationsschrift, Gießen, Justus-Liebig-Universität.
Claus, G., & Ebner, H. (1971). *Grundlagen der Statistik für Psychologen, Pädagogen und Soziologen.* Frankfurt a.M.-Zürich: Verlag Harri Deutsch.
Davis, G.C., Buchsbaum, M.S., & Bunney, W.E. (1978). Naloxone decreases diurnal variation in pain sensitivity and somatosensory evoked potentials. *Life Sci., 23,* 1449—1460.
Dhopesh, V.P., Herring, C.L., & Anwar, R. (1980). Tension headache in emergency department patients. *Psychosom., 21,* 631—635.
Dixon, W. J., Brown, M.B., Engelman, L., Frane, J.W., Hill, M.A., Jennrich, R.I., & Toporek, J.D. (1983). *BMDP statistical software: 1983. Printing with additions.* Berkeley: University of California Press.
Friedman, A.P., Finley, K.H., Graham, J.R., Kunkle, F.C., Ostfeld, A.M., & Wolff, H.G. (1962). Classification of headache. *Archives of Psychology, 6,* 173—176.
Glynn, C.J., & Floyd, J.W. (1976). The diurnal variation in perception of pain. *Proc. Roy. Soc. Med., 69,* 369—373.
Harper, R.G., & Steger, J.C. (1978). Psychological correlates of frontalis EMG and pain in tension headache. *Headache, 18,* 215—218.
Haynes, S.N., Griffin, P., Mooney, D., & Parise, M. (1975). Electromyographic biofeedback and relaxation instructions in the treatment of muscle contraction headaches. *Behav. Ther., 6,* 672—678.
Howarth, E. (1965). Headache, personality and stress. *Brit. J. Psychiat., 111,* 1193—1197.
Lille, F., & Cheliout, F. (1982). Variations in diurnal and nocturnal waking state in air traffic controllers. *Eur.J. Appl. Physiol., 49,* 319—328.

Lippold, O.C.J. (1967). Electromyography. In P.H. Venables & I. Martin (Eds.), *A manual of psychophysiological methods* (pp. 245—297). Amsterdam: North Holland.

Luria, R.E. (1975). The validity and reliability of the visual analogue mood scale. *J. Psychiat. Res., 12,* 51—57.

Marschall, P. (1983). *Differentielle Belastungs-/Beanspruchungsprozesse in leistungsfordernden Situationen in der Schule. Eine psychophysiologische Feldstudie.* Dissertation, University of Ulm.

Martin, P.R., & Mathews, A.M. (1978). Tension Headaches. Psychophysiological investigation and treatment. *J. Psychosom. Res., 22,* 389—399.

Ohnhaus, E.E., & Adler, R.(1975). Methodological problems in the measurement of pain: A comparison between the verbal rating scale and the visual analogue scale. *Pain, 1,* 379—384.

Philips, C. (1977). A psychological analysis of tension headache. In S. Rachman (Ed.), *Contributions to medical psychology, Vol. 1* (pp. 91—113). Oxford: Pergamon Press.

Philips, C. (1978). Tension headache. Theoretical problems. *Behav. Res. Ther., 16,* 249—261.

Philips, C., & Hunter, M.S. (1982). *A psychophysiological investigation of tension headache.* Unpublished manuscript.

Pöllmann, L., & Hildebrandt, G. (1979). Circadian variations of potency of placebos on pain threshold in healthy teeth. *Chronobiological, 6,* 145.

Pozniak-Patewicz, E. (1976). "Cephalgic" spasm of head and neck muscles. *Headache, 15,* 261—266.

Procacci, P. (1972). Änderungen der Schmerzschwelle für Hautstiche während des Tages- und Monatsrhythmus. In R. Janzen & W.-D. Keidel (Eds.), *Internationales Symposium über den Schmerz, Rottach-Egern 1969* (pp. 47—50). Stuttgart: Thieme.

Rugh, J.D. (1979). Clinical research in behavioral dentistry. In *Proceedings of the 2nd National Conference on Behavioral Dentistry.* Morgantown, West Virginia, West Virginia University, October 8—9.

Rugh, J.D., & Solberg, W.K. (1976). Psychological implications in temporomandibular pain and dysfunction. *Oral Sci. Rev., 7,* 3—30.

Schlote, B.M. (1987). *Psychophyiologische Feldstudie zum Spannungskopfschmerz.* Ulm: PSZ-Verlag.

Simons, D.J., Day, C., Goodell, H., & Wolff, H.G. (1943). Experimental studies on headache: Muscles of the scalp and neck as sources of pain. *Res. Nervous Ment. Diseases, 23,* 228—245.

Sweetman, B.J., Page, S., McMaster, G.W., Ellam, S., & Anderson, J.A.D. (1980). EMG correlates of low back pain work factor observations. In F.D. Stott, E.B. Raftery & L. Goulding (Ed.), *ISAM 1979: Proceedings of the third international symposium on ambulatory monitoring* (pp. 434—443). London-New York-Toronto-Sydney-San Francisco: Academic Press.

Traue, H.C., Bischoff, C., & Zenz, H. (1981). EMG-Unterschiede bei Personen mit und ohne Kopfschmerzen in einer sozialen Belastungssituation. In W. Michaelis (Ed.), *Bericht über den 32. Kongreß der DGfPs in Zürich 1980* (pp. 742—745). Göttingen: Hogrefe.

Traue, H.C., Gottwald, A., Henderson, P.R., & Bakal, D.A. (1985). Nonverbal expressiveness and activity in tension headache sufferers and controls. *I. Psychosom Res. 29,* 375—381.

Travell, J. (1952). Myofascial trigger points: Clinical review. In J.J. Bonica & D. Albe-Fessard (Ed.), *Advances in pain research and therapy, Vol. 1* (pp. 919—926). New York: Raven Press.

Travell, J. (1976). Myofascial trigger points: Clinical review. In J.J. Bonica & D. Albe-Fessard (Eds.), *Advances in pain research, Vol. 1* (pp. 919—926). New York: Raven Press.

Travell, J., & Rinzler, S.H. (1952). The myofascial genesis of pain. *Post. Grad. Med., 9*, 425—434.

Tunis, M.M., & Wolff, H.G. (1954). Studies of headache: Cranial artery vasoconstruction and muscle contraction headache. *Arch. Neurol. Psychiatry, 71*, 425—434.

Wolf-Cramer, B. (1984). Zum Problem der Diagnostik von Spannungskopfschmerz. *Psychother. med. Psychol., 34*, 81—89.

Zipp, P. (1982). Recommendations for the standardization of lead positions in surface electromyography. *Eur. J. Appl. Physiol., 50*, 41—54.

Myogenic Factors in Low Back Pain

Roland Teufel and Harald C. Traue

This chapter reviews the hypotheses of dysfunctional muscular activity as a cause for low back pain from a theoretical and empirical point of view. Different etiological models for low back pain from dynamic psychology, family therapy, and behavioral theory are presented. In respect to the differential diagnostic problems it is shown that possibly every model can be applied to a certain subgroup of patients. All theoretical models postulate a somatic disposition or a sensibility to develop pain in the lower back for their patients.

The behavioral low back pain models are based on several assumptions concerning the muscle tension reactions: higher paraspinal resting levels, higher paraspinal EMG during various postures and movements, greater reactivity in the muscular system under stress, and a simultaneous reduction of tension and pain under treatment. Empirical studies support heightened resting levels and a greater response under personally relevant stress conditions, while the investigation of movements and postures failed to differentiate between low back pain patients and pain-free controls. Although some treatment studies observe a reduction of tension and pain under biofeedback, these data did not prove a causal relationship between changes in the muscular activity and pain reduction. Finally conclusions for further research to develop better diagnostic procedures are made.

Epidemiology and Definition

Low back pain (LBP) causes great subjective suffering in patients and places a great economic burden on the health and insurance systems of a society. According to Glenn, Brown, Rhodes, and Lancourt (1981), 90% of all patients suffering less than two months will become pain-free with or without treatment. However, 50% of these patients will again suffer from back pain later in life. On the other hand, about 60% of all LBP patients who have the disease for more than 6 months will become chronically ill (Akerson, 1981), and 80% of these patients will become permanently work disabled. According to Horal (1969), the disease is most prevalent in the 40—60-year age group, affecting both men and women equally. Since this disability strikes long before retirement, it is not surprising that 18 billion US-dollars are spent anually on LBP treatment in addition to costs for rehabilitation, compensation payments, and other services (Haber, 1971). This estimate covers all back pain patients.

In the Federal Republic of Germany, 17% of all patients suffer from some kind of rheumatic disease (Miltner, Birbaumer, & Gerber, 1986), and according to Georg, Stuppardt, and Zoike, (1981), 10% of all work-related disabilities are caused by a spinal illness (data collected by German insurance companies in 1980). Moreover, it is a fact that bank employees below the age of 30 tend to suffer more from lumbago than do blue-collar workers. Thus, because of the shift from manual work to more and more office workplaces, a proportional increase of LBP can be expected.

Many physicians consider LBP an undiagnosable somatic disease since no specific causes can be determined. For a superficial classification it seems appropriate to describe Low Back Pain in a first step with what is *excluded* by the definition: such diseases as inflammatory back pain like chronic polyarthritis, spondylitis, etc., or degenerative processes like herniation of disc or pain as a result of lordosis, kyphosis, or skoliosis. The back pain we are referring to is pain in the lumbar region, where under certain (hypothetical) psychological circumstances muscular systems become affected by way of a dysfunctional regulatory mechanisms responsible for the aching area.

This low back pain is defined by the "Classification of Chronic Pain" (Merskey, 1986) as "Low Back Pain of Psychological Origin: Muscle Tension Pain" (Code 533.x7b) as virtually continuous pain in any part of the body due to sustained muscle contraction and provoked by emotional causes or by persistent overuse of particular muscles.

With this definition it becomes necessary to introduce etiological models for LBP developed in clinical psychology and behavioral medicine. The reported etiological models originate in psychoanalysis, family therapy, and mainly in learning and stress theory.

Etiological Models

Psychoanalysis

Psychoanalysis usually explains chronic back pain with the Freudian concept "conversion hysteria." According to this theory, intrapsychic conflicts are converted into a somatic illness in order to remain unconscious. Ahrens (1986) describes the personality of low back pain patients in the following manner: "chased, rigid, hyperactive and self-controlled." These character traits in combination with masochistic tendencies would cover-up the desire for "dependency" and "letting oneself go." Other psychoanalytic authors describe LBP patients as workaholic, unable to enjoy life, and having a compulsive social attitude. They are in constant rivalry with their siblings and peers, but demonstrate strong affections for children and other dependent people. Fleck's (1975) observations concerning LBP patients are as follows: LBP patients display feelings of rejection and worthlessness which have been with them since childhood. Labhardt (1976) focus on the following character traits: "fear of dependency," "acceptance of submission," "lack of self-confidence," and an "extrem dependency on praise."

Hanvik (1951) compared the MMPI profiles of LBP patients with a somatic diagnosis against those MMPI profiles of LBP patients without a somatic diagnosis (functional pain). The former had lower scores on the MMPI scales "hysteria" and "hypochondria" and higher scores on the "depression" scale than did the latter. However, patients with functional low back pain attained higher depression scores than the normal population. These results were described as a conversion "v."

Some empirical findings support the assumption that depression may be a cause for back pain (Lopez-Ibor, 1972; Kielholz, 1974). Further evidence is provided by the fact that antidepressive drugs successfully reduce somatic pain (Blumer, Heilbronn, Padraza, & Pope, 1980). However, Large (1980), Sternbach, Murphy, and Akerson, (1973), and Sternbach, Wolf, and Murphy (1973) are of a different opinion. On the basis of their positive correlations between depression and pain duration, they interpreted depression as a *consequence* of pain. Altogether one can conclude that psychoanalysis explains low back pain on a psychological basis while disregarding the biopsychological nature of pain processes in general and especially the relevance of dysfunctional muscle tension, which cannot be adequately explained by personality factors and psychodynamic terms. In addition, with the exception of the Freudian "conversion hysteria theory" (symptom = symbol of the unconscious conflict), the traditional dynamic personality hypotheses include no assumptions about the lumbar area as the body target of the conflict.

Family Therapy Theory

Minuchin (1974) developed a comprehensive model for psychosomatic diseases including LBP of particular family members. According to this model, LBP or other diseases are the result of a psychological disposition of that individual in combination with four transactional characteristics of the family members:
– overprotection,
– rigidity,
– emotional over-engagement,
– fear of conflicts.

Before having any symptoms mainly one child or one of several children of a particular family has the specific function of stabilizing the neurotic family constellation. With help of these specific interaction styles, a family homeostasis is established to avoid open conflicts. Minuchin argues that with such a constellation, it will only be a matter of time until the affected child develops some kind of psychosomatic illness. Moreover, the belief is that the weakest part of the body will exhibit the symptoms. Once the child has become ill, the other family members will increase their typical behavior. Such behavior on part of the family will of course lead to a reinforcement of the illness behavior (pain) and the symptoms (interpreted from a behavioral point of view). Finally, it has to be noted that no prospective study exists in family therapy research. Like depression, family characteristics can be seen as a consequence of the illness of a family member as well.

Behavioral Models

Operant conditioning model: While symptom reinforcement plays an important role in the above-described family theory, Fordyce's (1976) operant conditioning model focuses mainly on the learning of illness behavior. He assumes that an initially acute pain can lead to the chronification of pain if it has positive consequences for the individual or helps him or her to avoid negative consequences. It should be mentioned that there is a similarity between the operant conditioning model of pain and the dynamic conceptualization of "secondary gain of illness." In accordance with operant conditioning and family theory, Block, Kemper, and Gaylor (1980) demonstrated the social reinforcement of pain behavior by the spouses of LBP patients with methods of behavior observation. This result supports the role of social factors in the operant conditioning model. Anderson and Rehm (1984) found that pain intensity correlated with perceived "satisfaction in a relationship." Although the operant model is able to explain a considerable amount of variance of the chronification of LBP, it is rarely able to explain the onset of pain and the initial pain processes.

Classical conditioning model: Gentry and Bernal (1977) concluded from their studies that originally neutral stimuli are frequently contingent with elicited pain stimuli. Pain leads to heightened activity of the muscles in the affected area, and this increase in muscle activity subsequently leads to even more pain. Fear of pain makes the individual avoid physical activities, so that sensitization ensues. Thus, a pain-muscle tension-pain circle is established. Although one might get the impression that this paradigm may be overestimated, it is able to explain theoretically the initial onset and chronification of pain. Nevertheless, the classical conditioning model is rather simple and needs several additional assumptions: First, the afflicted body part is the pain-prone one; second, classical conditioned muscle tension leads to pain. It therefore makes more sense to consider this model as one possibility of a pain onset condition as well as an adequate explanation for certain subgroups of LBP sufferers.

Diathesis-Stress Models

A more comprehensive model for the explanation of LBP is the diathesis-stress model, derived from the work of Levi (1974). This model is based on the hypothesis of a predisposition of the body and persistent stressful events. In an influential work Flor (1984) has proposed a diathesis-stress model for low-back-pain patients. Her notion is that relevant personal stressors are able to overactivate the muscles in the lumbago region (m. erector trunci). Moreover, the inability to cope with this stress will lead to the permanent activation of the affected muscles and subsequently to ischemia and pain.

Mainly three conditions are necessary for the occurrence of a hyperactivation of the muscles in the lumbar region:

- the existence of a response stereotype reaction (diathesis) in the lumbar region;
- the existence of relevant personal stressful situations (either permanent or intermittent);
- the inability of the individual to cope with stress.

The possibilities of the interaction within the system of Flor are shown in Figure 1.

Bischoff and Traue (1983) offered a very similar but more complex multidimensional model for the etiology of myogenic headache which includes classical and operant conditioning, and can also be applied to low back pain of myogenic origin. The model consists of three seperate but related components:

- the physiological relationship between muscle tension and pain;
- the hypothesis of critically increased muscle activity;
- the conditioning of dysfunctional muscle activity.

The physiological relationships between tension, biochemical processes and pain and the circuit-like interactions are shown in Figure 2.

Most important for pain events are the possibilities of decreasing the threshold of mechanosensitive nociceptors by changing the biochemical milieu through long-term muscle activity which diminishes the available supply of oxygen, and consequently bradykinine, prostaglandine and serotonin become released. These substances not only lower the threshold of the nociceptors with regard to mechanical stimuli, they also tend to stimulate chemosensitive nociceptors. As a result, already moderate muscle contractions that can be induced by psychological stress may cause a considerable amount of pain.

Muscle pain is not necessarily associated with sustained contractions of the skeletal muscles. Like Flor, Turk, and Birbaumer (1985), the authors assume from their experimental pain research that increased muscle activity occurs mainly in particular stiuations of stress (personal and social), but also in situations of relief. Under stress conditions within a specific time period, the muscle activity can reach a critical point beyond which regenerative processes in the muscle physiology are no longer effective. While Flor postulates a general increase of muscle contractions Bischoff and Traue (1983) differentiate between five ideal situational patterns which add up to the so-called *critical amount of muscular activity*:

- heightened muscular activity in stressful situations;
- a prolonged reduction period of muscle activity following stressful situations;
- increased muscle tension in relief-type situations;
- muscle tension due to the accumulation of stressful situations-muscle tensions (see Figure 3) due to prolonged, particularly stressful situations.

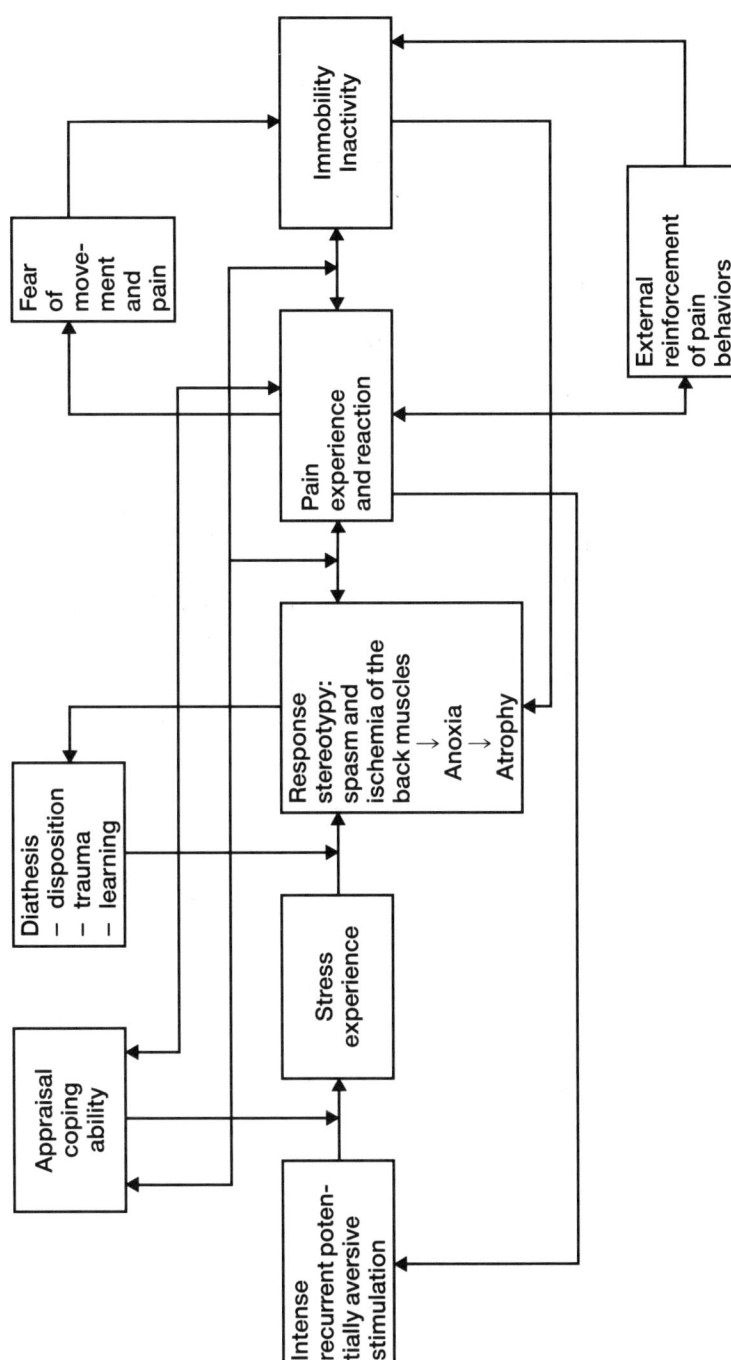

Figure 1. Diathesis-stress model for LBP by Flor (1985).

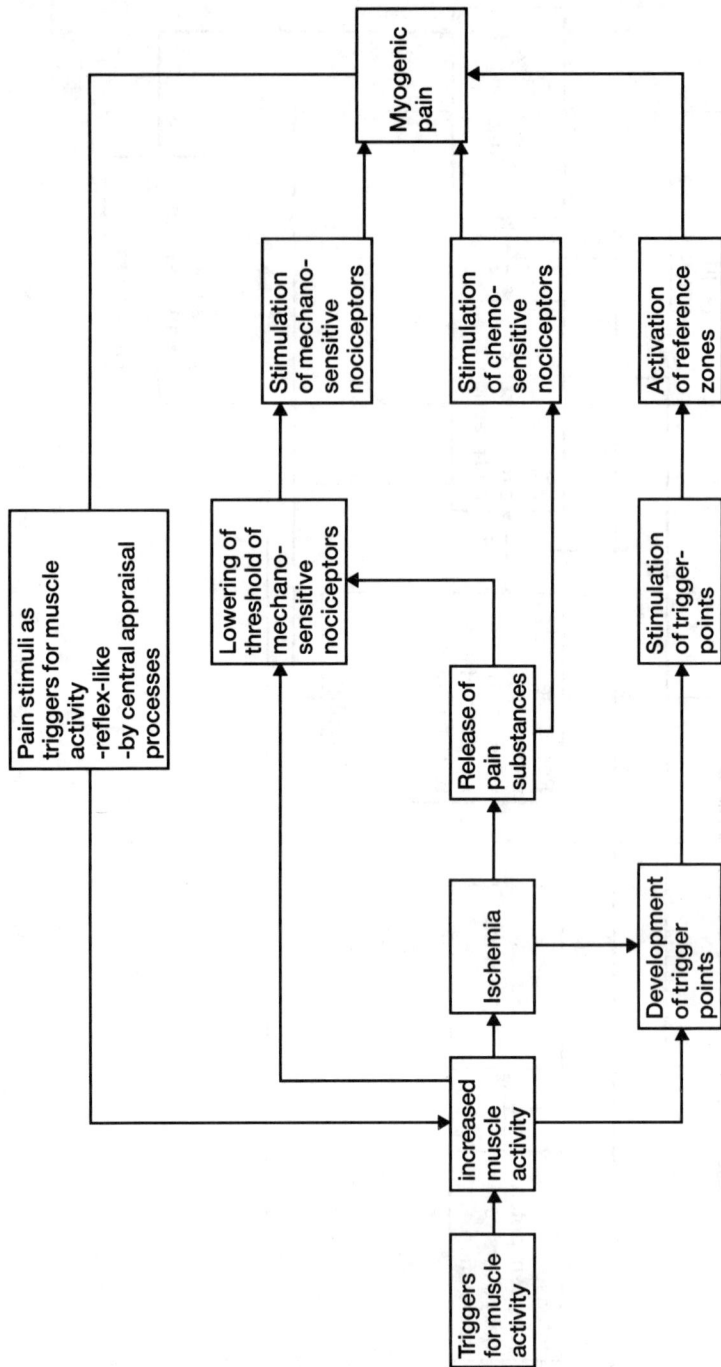

Figure 2. Physiology of myogenic pain (Bischoff & Traue, 1987).

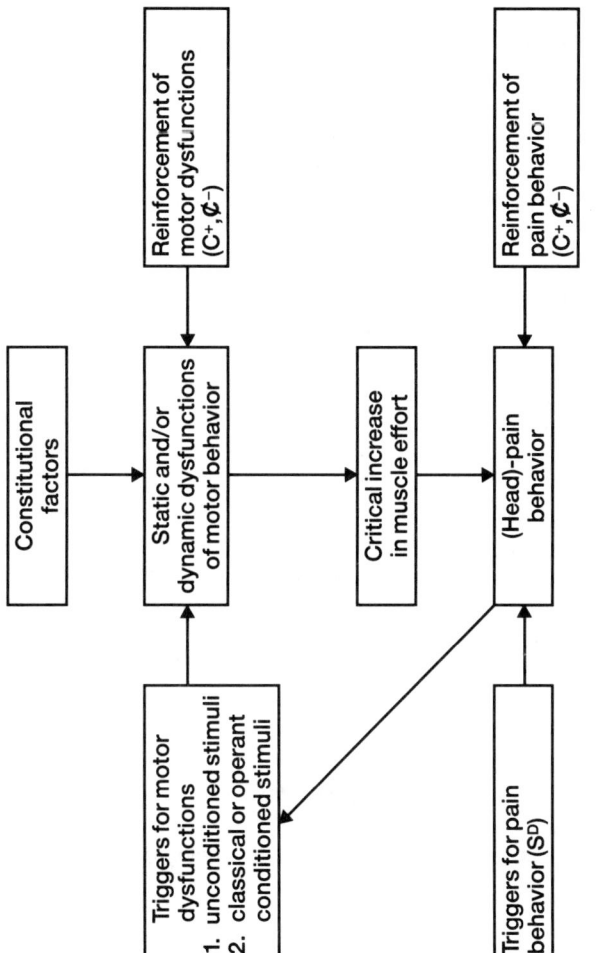

Figure 3. Simplified causal scheme for myogenic headache (Bischoff & Traue, 1983).

This model views muscle tension as behavior, comprising voluntary and reflexive motor acts and both governed by learning principles. The somewhat simplified model (the original version is published in Bischoff & Traue, 1983) puts the dysfunctional muscle tension at the center of the pain process and arranges the trigger and reinforcement conditions around it. The model extends the earlier model of Epstein and Cinciripini (1981) in as much as muscle dysfunctions are the main condition of a pain development.

Bischoff and Traue (1983) gave a very simplified but comprehensive example to explain their model: "Imagine a child who is repeatedly and unexpectedly beaten on his head by his parents. This child may develop myogenic headache when his parents are present in the same room. Then, his parents will have become conditioned stimuli eliciting heightened tension in the muscles of neck and shoulder. The unconditioned reflex, in this example consists of the pain-by-being-beaten-stimulus, which, as a reflex, leads to ducking the head (classical conditioning)."

Muscle tension increases may be modified by operant conditioning, when the corresponding voluntary motor acts are reinforced. To return to the child of their example: "A child when beaten is likely to exhibit a fight or flight reaction (Cannon, 1929). If the parents punish fight or flight behaviors, the child probably learns to inhibit these behaviors by negative reinforcement. Therefore, the motor impulses will endure and, combined with inhibitory behavior, cause dysfunctional muscle tension increases and prolonged recovery periods."

This does not mean that the authors negate the significance of different types of cognitive functions such as "coping with stress" or other constitutional factors. A complete presentation of all variables involved would not outline the causal scheme any better. Bischoff and Traue's model can therefore be seen as an elaborated diathesis-stress model based on the prevailing knowledge of pain processes. This model includes a great number of discrete behavioral possibilities available to the individual with which he or she can acquire myogenic pain.

Conclusion

The following conclusions can be drawn from the etiological models of low back-pain:

1. Most of the described models were not specifically developed for low back pain, but were applied to it. To date no model exists which is in total based on empirical studies.

2. Most empirical studies are generally retrospective. The chronification process—which a comprehensive model is supposed to describe—cannot be represented by such a procedure.

3. One can assume that these models are valid for specific subgroups of LBP patients.

4. All models are based on the assumption of a specific somatic disposition and pain proneness. A purely psychological etiology in the sense of conversion hysteria probably pertains to only a small percentage of patients.

Empirical Evidence of Myogenic Factors in LBP

All described etiolgical models try to explain low back pain in terms of their theoretical systems. Especially in models based on learning theory and/or stress theory do the myogenic factor plays a prominent role. To estimate the influence of this factor, a great number of investigations have been carried out in the past two decades.

As could be expected, this empirical literature presents a contradictory picture. A comprehensive review can be found in the theoretical study from Nouwen and Bush (1984). Based on the different behavioral models currently in existence, they derived the following hypotheses:

1. The resting paraspinal EMG will be higher in LBP patients than in pain-free controls.
2. The paraspinal EMG during various postures and movements will be higher in LBP patients than in pain-free controls.
3. Paraspinal EMG in LBP patients will be more reactive to stress than pain-free controls
4. The reduction of paraspinal EMG correlates with a pain reduction in LBP patients.
5. While paraspinal EMG will be elevated in LBP patients, other muscle groups will show normal EMG levels both at rest and as a response to stress.

The authors conclude that at the best only 50% of the investigated studies could confirm these hypotheses. We will now shortly report the main studies in respect of these five hypotheses.

Hypothesis I: The resting paraspinal EMG will be higher in LBP patients than in pain-free controls (Table 1).

Of the 11 investigations surveyed, 7 support the hypothesis that the resting paraspinal EMG will be higher in LBP patients than in pain-free controls. Kraft, Johnson, and Laban (1968) came to the result that resting muscles showed EMG silence in all cases. But it should be noted that they sampled 29 fibrositis (and not LBP) patients and used needle electrodes, where just a few number of muscle fibres are represented in the EMG. It was Cobb, de Vries, Urban, Luekens, and Bagg (1975) who found differences in EMG levels with surface electrodes, but not with needle electrodes (induced pain situations and pain-free situations).

In spite of the fact that most studies support the hypothesis, the contradictory results of Kraft, Johnson, and Laban (1968), Kravitz, Moore, and Glaros,(1981), and Collins, Cohen, Naliboff, and Schandler (1982) may be due to assessment procedures: Patients were instructed, to relax in order to create a stress-free setting for the investigation. Under this condition the probability of stress-related increased muscle tension is minimal.

Table 1. The resting paraspinal EMG will be higher in LBP-patients than in pain-free controls.

authors	patients	type of electrodes	measuring site	instruments	conditions/findings
Arrayo (1966)	20 patients with back and myofibrisitis pain	needle electrodes	fibrostic modules	—	increased EMG in prone position with muscles relaxed
Awad (1973)	10 patients with myofibrositis	needle electrodes	trapezius, triceps and quadriceps muscles	—	while resting EMG for 6 out of 10 patients
Cobb et al. (1975)	7 patients with induced pain	surface and needle electrodes	PSM* (paraspinal muscle)	gain setting 10 u v/cm integrated EMG	resting muscles showed increased EMG with surface electrodes but not with needles
Collins et al. (1982)	11 LBP patients 11 pain free controls	surface electrodes	PSM, 2 cm lateral to L_{3-4}	—	no difference while standing
Cram & Steger (1983)	9 LBP patients 41 controls	surface electrodes	PSM at T_1, T_6, T_{10}, L_3	integrated EMG (2 sec.)	while sitting and standing no EMG differences but side-asymmetries in lumbar area
de Vries (1966)	15 subjects with exercise induced pain	surface electrodes	elbow-flexors	integrated EMG	increased EMG with resting muscles
de Vries (1968)	8 LBP patients 4 controls	surface electrodes	PSM at L_1-L_5	integrated EMG (1 min)	of those who developed pain EMG increased; those who developed no pain EMG same as controls
Elliot (1944)	14 patients with sciatica	surface electrodes	tender areas in sciatica nerve distribution	—	resting muscles showed increased EMG for 8 of 14
Jayasinghe et al. (1978)	7 LBP patients 4 controls	surface electrodes	PSM at L_4-L_5	integrated EMG	increased EMG for LPB patients compared with controls

Table 1 (Continued).

authors	patients	type of electrodes	measuring site	instruments	conditions/findings
Kraft et al. (1968)	29 fibrositis patients	needle electrodes	PSM	gain setting 100 m V/ division	resting muscles showed EMG silence in all cases
Kravitz et al. (1981)	22 LBP patients 17 normals	surface electrodes	lumbar PSM	integrated EMG	no difference in resting muscles between LBP and normals

* PSM = Paraspinal muscle

Table 2. The paraspinal EMG during various posture and movements will be higher in LBP patients than in pain-free controls.

authors	patients	type of electrodes	measuring site	instruments	conditions/findings
Collins et al. (1982)	11 BP patients 11 controls	surface electrodes	PSM* 2 cm lateral L_3–L_4	—	while moving EMG LBP patients lower than controls
Hoyt et al. (1981)	40 LBP patients 40 controls	surface electrodes	PSM and RAM*	integrated EMG	higher EMG asymmetry for BP patients in various postures
Price et al. (1948)	BP patients (no. not reported)	surface electrodes	PSM	—	During head turning mild increase in upper back EMG; for head raising moderate increase in upper back and mild increase in lower back
Wolf & Basmajian (1978)	9 LBP patients 66 normals	surface electrodes	PSM at L_{3-4}	integrated EMG (10 sec)	during various dynamic movements LBP patients EMG lower than controls

* RAM = Rectus abdomen muscles, * PSM = paraspinal muscle

In summary, there is some empirical evidence in the literature for a sustained increase in muscle tension in LBP patients, which disappear under relaxation.

Hypothesis II: The paraspinal EMG during various postures and movements will be higher in LBP patients than in pain-free controls (Table 2).

In Price, Clare, and Ewerhardt (1948) and Wolf, Basmajian, Russe, and Kutner (1979) there is no support for this hypothesis. In fact Collins et al. (1982), Wolf and Basmajian (1978), and Hoyt et al. (1981) found that during various movements the EMG of LBP patients is even lower than in controls. Side asymmetries are increasingly thought to play an important role in the diagnosis of low back syndromes (Cram & Steger, 1983).

Furthermore, there exists a different approach to the etiology of low back pain advocated by Basmajian (1978), Wolf and Basmajian, (1978), and Collins et al.(1982). Their understanding of LBP is based on the biomechanical effects of faulty neuromuscular activity. Faulty patterns of muscular activity are responsible for side asymmetries and abnormally low levels of paraspinal muscle activity. This kind of innervation allows the spine in dynamic movements to become instable and irritate nerve endings by compression, and results in mechanically induced pain.

Hypothesis III: Paraspinal EMG in LBP patients will be more reactive to stress than pain-free controls (Table 3).

There is empirical evidence for the conclusion that personally neutral stressors like "mental arithmetic" or "cold pressor test" are unable to induce enough stress and subsequently to increase paraspinal activity (Flor, 1984). With respect to the pain target of LBP, some biological specifications which separate the somatic control of back muscles compared to other muscle groups should not be forgotten. The muscles of the erector trunci are quite special indeed, since they are innervated in a unique fashion: Each individual segment of the back is innervated seperately. This kind of segmental innervation is usually found in old phylogenetic structures (e.g., like those of the earthworm). The electrical activity on these muscles can only be brought to a complete standstill during deep general anesthesia. It seems that human back muscles possess a morphologic structure that is particularly suited to elicit biologically determined responses (like flight-fight, Cannon, 1929). The inability to cope with stress is viewed as a necessary condition for the occurrence of hyperactivation of the muscles in the lumbar region. But it is important to note that stressors have to be experienced as personally relevant (Flor, 1985) in order to elicit muscle tension responses. In the early times of mankind, this type of arousal was generally caused by frightening events. At present most of these bodily reactions are elicited by the appraisal of aversive situations.

Table 3. Paraspinal EMG in LBP patients will be more reactive to stress than of pain-free controls.

authors	patients	type of EMG-	stressors	results
Holmes & Wolf (1952)	65 LBP patients	needle electrodes	stress interview	increased paraspinal muscle activity (no quantification)
Collins et al. (1982)	11 LBP patients 11 controls	surface electrodes	cold pressure mental arithmetic	no statistically significant group differences
Flor et al. (1985)	17 LBP patients 17 general pain patients 17 controls	surface electrodes	discussion of personal stress and pain, mental arithmetic, reciting the alphabet	increased EMG (PSM) and delayed return to baseline (for LBP patients) as a reaction of personal relevant stressors (no difference for neutral stressors)
Cohen et al. (1986)	13 LBP patients	surface electrodes	cold pressure mental arithmetic	no difference between groups within various postures
Grabel (1973)	30 LBP patients 30 controls	—	expectation of electric shock and relaxation	LBP patients show higher EMG level independent of the stress condition and relaxation

Hypothesis IV: The reduction of paraspinal EMG correlates with a pain reduction in LBP patients (Table 4).

Studies testing the hypothesis that a reduction of muscle activity leads to a reduction of pain have resulted in contradictory findings. In most of these biofeedback studies, patients reduced their EMG levels and decreased their pain. Although the biofeedback treatment is successful in pain and tension reduction, there are doubts as to whether or not the motor learning is the main factor for pain reduction. From the data base of these studies, one can conclude that this hypothesis is confirmed—at least for therapy effects.

Unfortunately, most of the studies report no follow-up of EMG data, although Nouwen and Solinger (1979) did observe an increase in muscle tension, the pain

Table 4. The reduction of paraspinal EMG correlates with pain reduction in LBP patients.

authors	patients	site	sessions	procedure	results	follow up
Belar & Cohen (1979)	1 LBP patient (71 years)	shoulder	5 baseline 1 relaxation 17 biofeedback	1) baseline 2) relaxation 3) biofeedback	decrease of EMG level and pain	EMG and pain reduction after 6 weeks
Freeman et al. (1980)	8 men	PSM*	50 reduction from baseline max. 10 sessions	baseline followed by biofeedback	4 reached criterion and reduced pain, 2 did not, but reduced pain, 2 did not and no pain reduction	after 3 months those who reached criteria maintained pain reduction
Flor et al. (1986)	24 BP patients	pain site	12 sessions BP BL-biofeedback-	group I (8 patients) and pain only for BL in prone position sitting and standing, group II (8-patients) pseudotherapy, group III (11 patients) medical treatments	decrease of EMG and pain only for group I	after 4 months offset maintained
Keefe et al. (1981)	111 mixed diagnostic types	frontalis upper trapezius	10 BF sessions in mean	EMG biofeedback, relaxation, medication reduction, physical therapy	decreased pain and medication use	—
Large & Lamb (1983)	18 patients with musculo-skeletal pain	pain site, from frontalis if pain generalized	6 BF sessions	Three conditions: 1) waiting list 2) BF given at very low gain 3) EMG BF given for decreased activity	decreased EMG and pain	—

Table 4. (Continued). The reduction of paraspinal EMG correlates with pain reduction in LBP patients.

authors	patients	site	sessions	procedure	results	follow up
Nigl & Fisher-Williams (1980)	4 LBP patients	unilateral PSM* over pain site	15 BF sessions in mean	EMG biofeedback and imagery techniques	decreased EMG and pain	after 3 months effect maintained only for 1 of 4
Nouwen & Solinger (1979)	19 LBP patients 7 controls (waiting list)	across PSM near 2nd lumbar vertebra	20 sessions (45 min.)	1) baseline 2) EMG biofeedback during movement and rest	EMG and pain reduction	after 4 months effect maintained
Nouwen (1983)	20 LBP patients	PSM at L_{4-5}	15 sessions	1) baseline 2) biofeedback 3) baseline	EMG decrease but no decrease in pain	—
Peck & Kraft (1977)	8 patients with back and shoulder pain	trapezius and PSM	10 BF sessions	EMG biofeedback training in tension perception	moderate decrease in EMG but no change in pain	—

* PSM = paraspinal muscle

remaining low. One can conclude from this that tension reduction decreases the pain but is not necessary for the maintenance of a pain-free state. In addition, one can assume that other therapeutic effects like a better stress management, a change in efficiency, and mobilization are powerful "sideeffects" of a biofeedback treatment.

Hypothesis V: While paraspinal EMG will be elevated in LBP patients, other muscle groups will show normal EMG levels both at rest and as a response to stress.

Sainsbury and Gibson (1954) reported that neither forearm nor frontalis EMG was higher in 17 LBP patients and in 30 pain-free controls. In addition, Collins et al. (1982) did not find group differences in patients and controls during baseline measurement in frontalis EMG. Unfortunately, neither Sainsbury and Gibson nor Collins et al. tested EMG differences from several placements within the LBP group. Similarly, Cram and Steger(1983) found generally only slight EMG differences within 11 placements (frontalis, lumbar, trapezius, etc.) in a group of 9 LBP patients, though they did not test these differences statistically. Thus, these studies are not designed to confirm hypothesis V.

Resumee

Most of the theoretical LBP models view muscle tension as a main factor in the physiological base of this disease. As a result of these myogenic low back pain models, the recently published pain classification defines a subgroup of low back pain as "LBP of psychological origin, type tension" caused by muscular hyperactivity as a consequence of psychological stress. Despite this definition, the empirical data supporting the myogenic model are weak. Only half of the studies found significant differences with respect to muscle tension activity.

There are, however, several problems regarding the empirical studies. First, the unsolved problem of a proper diagnosis. Normally, LBP is diagnosed by exclusion. EMG scanning methods are still in being explored and do not take social or natural stressors into account, although particularly these personally relevant stress conditions are important. The EMG measurements are too simplistic. It seems necessary to study change scores, recovery rates, and muscle patterns.

Second, not much is known about the psychological processes that are responsible, such as moderator variables like coping style, social support, or abilities to manage stress. There are no studies connecting these varaibles to the pain-tension-pain circle.

Finally, most of the retrospective studies are difficult to interpret, since the pain process itself might be responsible for behavior changes or even the observed EMG differences. Therefore, prospective studies are necessary to identify and separate physiological and psychological factors in the chronification of low back pain.

References

Ahrens,S. (1986). Chronische Lumbo-Ischialgie: Der Kranke nimmt sich zu scharf an die Kandarre. *Ärztliche Praxis, 43,* 1514—1517.

Akerson, K.M. (1981). Prediction of chronicity in low back patients. *Dissertation Abstracts International, 42,* 2513.

Anderson, L.P. & Rehm, L.P. (1984). The relationship between strategies of coping and perception of pain in three chronic pain groups. *Journal of Clinical Psychology, 40,* 1170—1177.

Arrayo, P. (1966). Electromyography in the evaluation of reflex muscle spasm. *Journal of Florida Medical Association, 53,* 29—31.

Awad, E.A. (1973). Interstitial myofibrositis: Hypothesis of the mechanism. *Archives of Physical Medicine and Rehabilitation, 54,* 449—453.

Basmajian, J.V. (1978). Cyclobenzaprine hydrochloriade effects on skeletal muscle spasm in the lumbar region and neck: Two double-blind controlled clinical and laboratory studies. *Archives of Physical Medicine and Rehabilitation, 59,* 58—63.

Belar, C.D., & Cohen, J.L. (1979). The use of EMG feedback and progressive relaxation in the treatment of a woman with chronic back pain. *Biofeedback and Self-Regulation, 4,* 345—353.

Bischoff, C., & Traue, H.C. (1983). Myogenic Headache. In K.A. Holroyd, B. Schlote & H. Zenz (Eds.), *Perspectives in research on headache* (pp. 66—90). Toronto/Lewiston, NY: C.J. Hogrefe.

Bischoff, C. & Zenz, H.,& Traue, H.C. (1986). Primärer Kopfschmerz. In Th. v. Uexküll (Ed.), *Psychosomatische Medizin* (3. Auflage, pp. 565—582). München: Urban & Schwarzenberg.

Bischoff, C., & Traue, H.C. (1987). Myogenic Headache: Theoretical considerations and empirical support. In J.P. Dauwalder, M. Perrez & V. Hobi (Eds.), *Controversial issues in behavior modification.* Amsterdam: Swets & Zeitlinger

Block, A., Kemper, E., & Gaylor, M.(1980). Behavioral treatment of chronic pain behavior: The spouse as a discriminative cue for pain behavior. *Pain, 9,* 243—252.

Blumer, D., Heilbronn, M., Padraza, E., & Pope, G.(1980). Systematic treatment of chronic pain with antidepressants. *Henry Ford Hospital Medical Journal, 28,* 15—21.

Cannon, W.B. (1929). *Bodily changes in pain, hunger, fear and rage.* New York: Appleton, Century.

Cobb,C.R., de Vries, H.A., Urban, R.T. Luekens, C.A., & Bagg, R.J.(1975). Electrical activity in muscle pain. *American Journal of Physical Medicine, 54,* 80—87.

Cohen, M.J., Swanson, G.A., Naliboff, B.D., Schandler, S.L., & McArthur, D.L. (1986). Comparison of electromyographic response patterns during postures and stress tasks in chronic low back pain patterns and control. *Journal of Psychosomatic Research, 30*(2), 135—141.

Collins, G.A., Cohen, M.J., Naliboff, B.D., & Schandler, S.L. (1982). Comparative analysis of paraspinal and frontalis EMG, heart rate and skin conductance in chronic low back pain patients and normal to various postures and stress. *Scand. Journal of J.Rehab. Med., 14,* 39—46.

Cram, J.R., & Steger, J.C. (1983). EMG scanning in the diagnosis of chronic pain. *Biofeedback and Self-Regulation, 8,* 229—241.

deVries, H.A. (1968). Quantitative electromyographic investigation of the spasm theory of muscle pain. *American Journal of Physical Medicine, 45,* 119—134.

deVries, H.A. (1966). Electromyographic fatigue curves in postural muscles, a possible etiology for idiopathic low back pain. *American Journal of Physical Medicine, 47,* 175—181.

Elliot, F.A. (1944). Tender muscles in sciatica. *Lancet, 1,* 47—49.

Epstein, L.H., & Cinciripini, P.M. (1981). Behavioral control of tension headaches. In J.M. Ferguson & C.B. Taylor (Eds.), *The comprehensive handbook of behavioral medicine*, Vol. 2. New York: Jamaica.

Fleck, H.C. (1975). Über psychodynamische Faktoren bei Wurzelreizerscheinungen. *Zeitschrift für Psychosomatik und Medizin, 21,* 118—128.

Flor, H. (1984). *Empirical evaluation of a diathesis-stress model of chronic back pain.* Dissertation, Universität Tübingen.

Flor, H., Turk, D.C., & Birbaumer, N. (1985). Assessment of stress-related psychophysiological reactions in chronic back pain patients. *Journal of Consulting and Clinical Psychology, 53*(3), 354—364.

Flor, H., Haag, G., & Turk, D.C. (1986). Long-term efficacy of EMG biofeedback for chronic rheumatic back pain. *Pain, 27,* 195—202.

Fordyce, W.E. (1976). *Behavioral methods for chronic pain and illness.* St. Louis: Mosby.

Freeman, C.W., Calsyn, D.A., Paige, A.B., & Halar, E.M. (1980). Biofeedback with low back pain patients. *American Journal of Clinical Biofeedback, 3,* 118—122.

Gentry, W.D., & Bernal, G.A.A. (1977). Chronic pain. In R.B. Williams & W.D. Gentry (Eds.), *Behavioral approaches to medical treatment.* Cambridge, MA: Ballinger.

Georg, A., Stuppardt, R., & Zoike, E. (1981). *Krankheit und arbeitsbedingte Belastungen, Bd.1.* Essen: Bundesverband der Betriebskrankenkassen.

Glenn, W.V., Brown, B.M., Rhodes, M.L., & Lancourt, J.E. (1981). Computerized body tomography and evaluation of lumbosacral spinal disease. In B.E. Finneson (Ed.), *Low back pain* (2nd ed.). London: Lippicott.

Grabel, J.A. (1973). Electromyographic study of low back muscle tension in subjects with and without chronic low back pain. *Dissertation Abstract, 34*(6-8), 2929—2930.

Haber, L.D. (1971). Disabling effects of chronic disease and impairment. *Journal of Chronic Disease, 24,* 469—487.

Hanvik, L.J. (1951). MMPI-Profiles in patients with low back pain. *Journal of Consulting Psychology, 15,* 350—353.

Holmes, Th.H., & Wolff, H.G. (1952). Life situations, emotions and backache. *Psychosomatic Medicine, 14,* 18—33.

Horal, J. (1969). The clinical appearance of low back disorders in the city of Gothenburg, Sweden. *Acta Orthop. Scand., 118,* 8—79.

Hoyt, W.H., Hunt, H.H., Depauw, M.A., Bard, D., Shaffer, F., Passias, J.N., Pobbins, D.H., Runyon, D.G., Semrad, S.E., Symonds, J.T., & Watt, K.C. (1981). Electromyographic assessment of chronic low back pain syndrome. *Journal of American Osteopathic Association, 80,* 728—730.

Jayasinghe, W.J., Harding, R.H., Anderson, J.A.D., & Sweetman, B.J. (1978). An electromyographic investigation of postural fatigue in low back pain. *Electromyography and Clinical Neurophysiology, 18,* 191—198.

Keefe, F.J., Black, A.R., Williams, R.B., & Surwit, R.S. (1981). Behavioral treatment of chronic low back pain: Clinical outcome and individual differences in pain relief. *Pain, 11,* 221—231.

Kielholz, R. (1974). *Masked depression.* Bern, Stuttgart, Wien: Hans Huber.

Kraft, G.H., Johnson, E.W., & Laban, M.M. (1968). The fibrositis syndrome. *Archives of Physical Medicine and Rehabilitation, 49,* 155—162.

Kravitz, E., Moore, M.E., & Glaros, A.G. (1981). Muscle activity in chronic low back pain. *Archives of Physical Medicine and Rehabilitation, 62,* 172—176.

Labhardt, A.(1976). *Psychosomatische und psychodynamische Aspekte weichteilrheumatischer Erkrankungen.* Referat: 17. Tagung der Deutschen Gesellschaft für Rheumatologie, Regensburg (unpublished observations).

Large, R.G. (1980). The psychiatrist and the chronic pain patient: 172 anecdotes. *Pain, 9,* 253—263.

Large, R.G., & Lamb, A.M. (1983). Electromyographic (EMG) feedback in chronic musculoskeletal pain: A controlled trial. *Pain, 17,* 167—177.

Levi, L. (1974). Psychosocial stress and disease: A conceptual model. In E.K. Gunderson & R.H. Rahe (Eds.), *Life stress and illness.* Springfield, IL: C.C. Thomas.

Lopez-Ibor, J.J. (1972). Masked depression. *British Journal of Psychiatry, 120,* 245—258.

Merskey, H. (1986). Classification of chronic pain. *Pain* (Suppl. 3). Amsterdam: Elsevier.

Miltner, W., Birbaumer, N., & Gerber, W.D. (1986). *Verhaltensmedizin.* Berlin: Springer-Verlag.

Minuchin, S. (1974). *Families and family therapy.* Cambridge, MA: Harvard University Press.

Nigl, A.J., & Fischer-Williams, M. (1980). Treatment of low back strain with electromyographic biofeedback and relaxation training. *Psychosomatics, 21,* 495—499.

Nouwen, A., & Bush, C. (1984). The relationship between paraspinal EMG and chronic low back pain. *Pain, 20,* 109—123.

Nouwen, A., & Solinger, J.W. (1979). The effectiveness of EMG biofeedback training in low back pain. *Biofeedback and Self-Regulation, 4,* 103—111.

Nouwen, A. (1983). EMG biofeedback used to reduce standing levels of paraspinal muscle tension in chronic low back pain. *Pain, 17,* 353—360.

Peck, C.L., & Kraft, G.H. (1977). Electromyographic biofeedback for pain related to muscle tension. *Archives of Surgery, 112,* 889—895.

Price, J.P., Clare, M.H., & Ewerhardt, F.H. (1948). Studies in low backache with persistent muscle spasm. *Archives of Physical Medicine, 29,* 703—709.

Sainsbury, P., & Gibson, J.G. (1954). Symptoms of anxiety and tension and the accompanying physiological changes in muscular systems. *J. Neurol. Neurosurg. Psychiat., 17,* 216—224.

Sternbach, R.A., Wolf, S.R., & Murphy, R.W. (1973). Aspects of chronic low back pain. *Psychosomatics, 14,* 226—229.

Sternbach, R.A., Murphy, R.W., & Akeson, W.H. (1973). Chronic low back pain: the "low-back loser."*Postgraduate Medicine, 53,* 135—138.

Wolf, S.L., & Basmajian, J.V. (1978). Assessment of paraspinal electromyographic activity in normal subjects and in chronic back pain patients using a muscle biofeedback device. In E. Asmussen, & K. Jorgensen (Eds.), *International series on biomechanics* (VIb, pp. 319—324). Baltimore, MD: University Park Press.

Wolf, S.L., Basmajian, J.V., Russe, T.C., & Kutner, M. (1979). Normative data on low back mobility and activity levels. *American Journal of Physical Medicine, 58,* 217—229.

SECTION B:
DIAGNOSTIC PROCEDURES

A Headache Interview

*Gabriele Manok and Helmuth Zenz**

We present a semi-standardized guide suited for conducting an initial interview with headache sufferers. The interview explores the characteristics of a headache attack, the conditions preceding and following it, and the psychosocial context it is embedded in. It also explores the patients' self-efficacy, their experience of their own body, their emotional processes as well as what they expect of the treatment. The interview enables the therapist to make clinical judgments about personality traits relevant to the treatment.

We examined the quality of clinical judgments using 35 videotaped interviews of headache sufferers. The inter-rater reliability of the judgments amounted to a mean value of 0.79. The judgments of the interviewing clinicians correlated with those of the clinicians observing the tape (mean value: 0.51). Two factor analyses of the "judgments by observers" matrix revealed the construct validity of the judgments.

Preliminary Note

With respect to psychogenic headache, fundamental research so far has not yet succeeded in answering elementary questions. For example, is it really necessary to classify migraine into various sub-groups such as: simple migraine, ophthalmic migraine, migraine accompagnée, basilary migraine, ophthalmophlegic migraine and other rather seldom occurring types (Gerber & Haag, 1982)? Or can we do without such a split-up as migraine is no autonomic syndrome, but rather together with tension headache forms a pathologic group (Bakal, 1982)? Is there a special tension headache as defined by the Ad Hoc Committee (Friedman, 1962) or is this just a label for all possible types of headache that are left over after a final exclusion (Philips, 1980)?

Considering such basic confusion the clinician might well sink into despair when trying to get material for a specific case. Clinical work, however, is generally governed by an overall objective as a result of its being part of a general concept of treatment. This overall concept is to be considered before an exact diagnosis is made and steps for a therapy concept are taken. We want to demonstrate this by showing you how our Department of Medical Psychology in Ulm, Germany, is involved with the treatment of a headache patient.

---

* Thanks to Marie-Luise Sefrin for her translation of the manuscript.

The Management of the Patient

The headache patient is usually referred by the family doctor to the Outpatient Pain Therapy Clinic, where about 150 headache patients per year are examined and treated. There the patient is then thoroughly examined. This examination includes recording a detailed medical history by an anesthesist. The examing doctor then refers the patient to certain departments of the University Clinic in Ulm, e.g., Neurology and ENT. In addition, important lab tests are carried out, an X-ray of the cervical spine is taken, and if necessary a cranial computer tomogram is also carried out (in case of suspicion of a tumor). The patient is then asked to come to the Pain Therapy Clinic for a second appointment. The doctor in charge of the case discusses these first results with the patient and explains the remaining examinations, including a psychological evaluation of the headache. At this time, the patient meets the liason psychologist from the Department of Medical Psychology of the Ulm University who is on duty in the Pain Therapy Clinic. The liason psychologist conducts a "warming up" discussion with the patient and orders further psychodiagnostics in our department. Before and after thus introductory discussion, the patient fills out various psychological tests, including a multidimensional pain scale, a medical complaint questionnaire, a biographical account, and two psychiatric scales. A clinician from the Department for Medical Psychology forms a clinical diagnostic interview with the patient. This discussion follows the interview guide presented in this paper. With informed consent from the patient, the conversation is filmed with a videocamera for research purposes. In addition, the psychologist forms an opinion about the patient's personality make-up with the use of a psychodiagnostic evaluation questionnaire included with the interview guide.

After this initial interview the patient fills out a detailed questionnaire which ascertains in a step-by-step form the patient's headache event and the factors that predominantly influence it. The therapist then writes a report for the Pain Therapy Clinic noting the test results and the findings of the headache questionnaire and of the interview. In a case study conference of the Therapy Clinic, all of the medical and psychological findings in question are discussed with the liason psychologist, and a joint therapy concept for the patient is formed. This concept is discussed with the patient in a further appointment.

Figure 1 shows the concept for the care given to the patient by the Pain Therapy Clinic.

Overall Objective

Most diagnostic procedures applied to headache patients take a course similar to that depicted above. In most cases the initial psychological interview with headache patients has above all a *consultation function*: It judges the patients who come to a medical institution seeking diagnostic clarification and therapy for

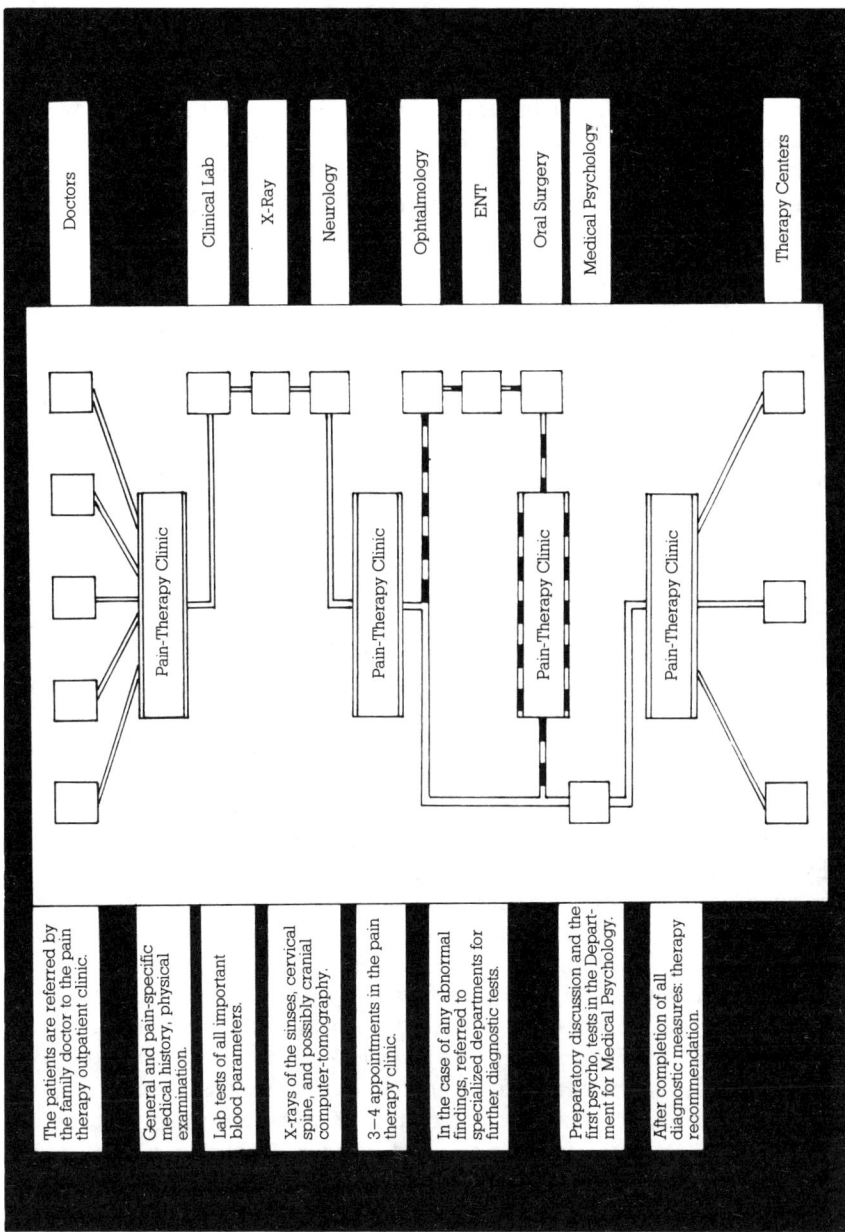

Figure 1. The process of managing the headache patient.

their headaches. The overall goal of the clinical discussion is to contribute to the general decision of how and whether the patient can be managed. This overall goal consists of various objectives, for example, determining the particular steps of treatment for a specific therapy form, or obtaining data for research. Aspects of care are considered, for example, whether social measures, such as a new job, appear relevant of realistic for the patient, whether the distance of the patient's residence from the medical institution plays a role, whether withdrawal therapy from analgesics is called for, or whether one type of therapy or another can be paid for by the patient's health insurance.

Though we could obtain all information required for such decisions by special questionnaires, we assume this would cause frustration and aggravation as most patients would miss an immediate contact to the psychologist. Questionnaires and tests are not suitable to satisfy the paient's demands for contact and communication. In addition, it is doubtful whether there exists any other method to obtain the information necessary for the understanding of the headache patient apart from conversation.

Methodological Aspect

The clinical tests used as a diagnostic instrument are usually found to be most reliable and objective. With respect to the patient, their diagnostic effect, however, is highly limited since they can only reflect a rather restricted aspect of a patient's behavior repertoire. Thus, the relevance of clinical diagnostic tests sometimes is rather questionable, the more so since, for these reasons, there is hardly any validity concerning the later establishment of a prognosis.

It is exactly because of these weak points that we presume the merits of a patient-oriented conversation as a diagnostic instrument. Not limited to the exact listing of objectively acquired data, the goal of such a method lies in *recognizing, understanding, and explaining* the subjective reality of the patient as an individual. When trying to get an idea about the complex personality make-up of a patient, not only is it important to the therapist what kind of things the patient mentions, but as well what the patient apparently does not (dare to) reveal. Here, the therapists also evaluates the patient's nonverbal behavior during the discussion. As a result of systematic inquiry and with emotional empathy for the individual personality, therapists can intensify their impressions, conceptions, and hypothesis about the patient's psychic and/or somatic problems. Through this discussion the doctor or psychologist is put in immediate contact with the patient and is able to experience all of the thoughts, feelings, aspects of behavior, and perceptions of the patient in both the present and past. This is why, under favorable conditions, a discussion in a positive atmosphere can result in more relevant statements concerning therapy and establishment of a prognosis that would be possible with the usual tests.

Concerning scientific principles such as objectivity, validity, and reliability, the findings obtained in an interview, however, are generally not satisfactory: Here is the decisive disadvantage of such a procedure.

An *interview procedure* may be considered as reliable:

- if the findings of the interview are basically not affected by situational influences;
- if repeated tests using this instrument within a time interval have produced identical findings.

Validity of an interview procedure is obtained

- if the procedure is able to gather the necessary information about the patient with the least possible distortion;
- if the findings of the interview positively correspond to the data acquired by other measuring techniques.

Bibliographical data as to reliability and validity of interview procedures vary considerably. Whereas Matarazzo (1965) talks about interview reliabilities of 0.49—0.81 and of validities of between 0.36 and 0.64, Guilford (1965) reports reliabilities of between 0.36 and 0.49 and validities of between 0.01 and 0.41.

Considering these statistical findings, any interviewing method at first sight seems to be a rather unscientific pastime, at least if compared to usual testing procedures which lead if not to important, to very reliable data. This, however, ignores the fact that we cannot compare a test, the goal of which is restricted to acquiring a few personal characteristics, to an interview procedure made up to solve a complex scope of tasks.

As proved by Cronbach and Gleser (1957), wide-range measuring instruments suitable to verifying a number of assumptions are marked by a relatively low validity, whereas improved psychometric quality results in a reduced measuring range. Clinical diagnostic interviews trying to make relevant statements concerning diagnosis, therapeutical concept and expected prognosis thus cannot be replaced by test batteries showing a very limited relevance.

The interview guide we would like to introduce in this paper was developed for diagnostic discussions with headache patients as a way out of this dilemma. So far we have tested it on about 150 headache patients who have come to initial psycho-diagnostic discussions.

Fundamental Psychosomatic Ideas about an Initial Interview for Headache Patients

As to the contents of the interview we were governed by the pathogenetic hypothesis formed by the Ulm Research Group on the occurrence of psychogenic headache. This hypothesis has to be seen not only from a mere scientific vantage point, but also as a method to collect the complaints of pain expressed by the individual patient and assemble them to a diagnostic concept integrating both pathophysiologic and psychodynamic aspects.

According to the theory on myogenic headache developed by the Ulm University Group (Bischoff, Zenz, & Traue, 1986), we assumed that, like in other psychosomatic diseases, the following four factors are usually present in persons who express primary headache:

- an individual overresponsiveness to stress;
- an insufficient capacity of the patient to cope with stress;
- as a result of the previous two factors, (pathologically) elevated values of the muscoloskeletal system, also in times in which the stressor is not present. In case of migraine the cranial blood vessels are involved as a physiological system.
- we consider it possible that headache patients due to their poor coping capacity remain in stress situations too long and too often.

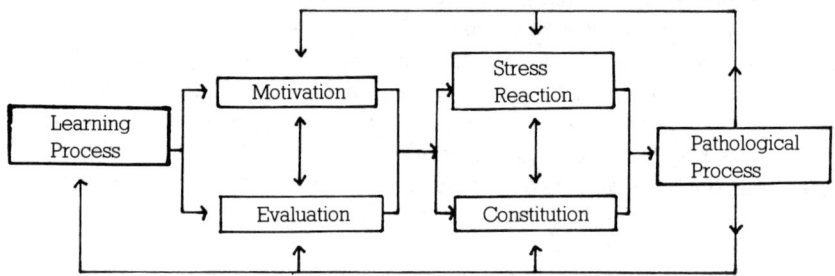

Figure 2. Psychosocial factors involved in a psychosomatic process.

In examining the origin of this patient make-up one can look to events and experiences in the patient's past. These experiences are the result of

- learning processes;
- their associated emotional cognitive evaluations, i.e., attitudes, expectation, suppositions;
- the motivational position with which a person deals with his or her environment.

For example someone who is strongly motivated and behaves in a "sensation-seeking" way (Zuckerman et al., 1964) will have more opportunities to develop strategies for managing the problems of daily life than someone who doesn't have these opportunities due to "stimulus-avoiding" behavior.

In addition, the length and duration of the stress reaction, i.e., the psychophysiologic reaction on stress is also determined by the special physical and psychic constitution of the patient. Chronicity of numerous and intensive stress reactions combined with constitutional facts finally leads to a pathological anatomic response. Just as, for example, the morphologically visible substrate of a constantly elevated arousal profile could be gastritis or a pancreatic ulcer, trigger points will form as a result of tension headache which are morphologically shown to be caused by degenerated muscle tissue.

Our concept is depicted in Figure 2.

The duration and frequency of stress situations is dependent on patients' cognitive situation analysis, their "evaluation" of immediate motivational processes, their accumulative primary or acquired coping skills, as well as the social situation in which the patients finds themselves. Frequency and duration of stress on their part provoke learning processes as an essential feedback element in an evaluation process. The combined action of these factors is shown in Figure 3.

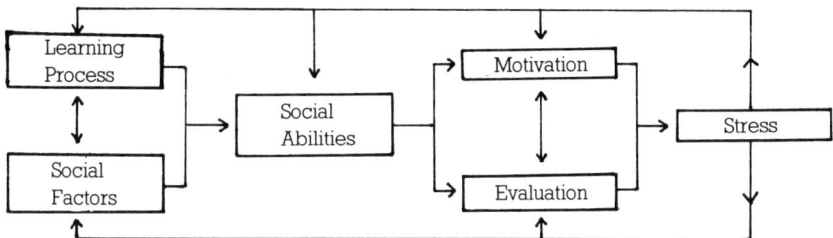

Figure 3. Psychosocial factors determining an enhanced stress reaction.

With respect to the genesis of headache, we proceed on the assumption that patients with chronic psychogenic headache are guided by way of acting toward emotional experiences, in which their perception of internal (introceptive) stimuli is either poorly integrated or not integrated at all. Figure 4 serves as an illustration. The feeling process of such headache patients occurs through the situation-dependent perception of external stimuli (path 1 and 7) more often than in people without headaches. In this case these patients are incapable or poorly capable of perceiving the accompanying physical effects that also occur at this time. The feeling process occurs then via paths 1, 2, 3, 7, and 8, but not via path 4, 5, and 6. Since internal stimuli are not well perceived, the physical peripheral reactions immediately produced by emotional challenge cannot be controlled and integrated while influencing body functions. Since the capability of an organism to perceive body signals correctly is an important adaptive function for survival, this deficiency causes hyper-reactions that induce acute pain attacks and, in case of chronicity, produce a general susceptibility to attack-prone situations. They also result in a pathological change in the respective organic sys-

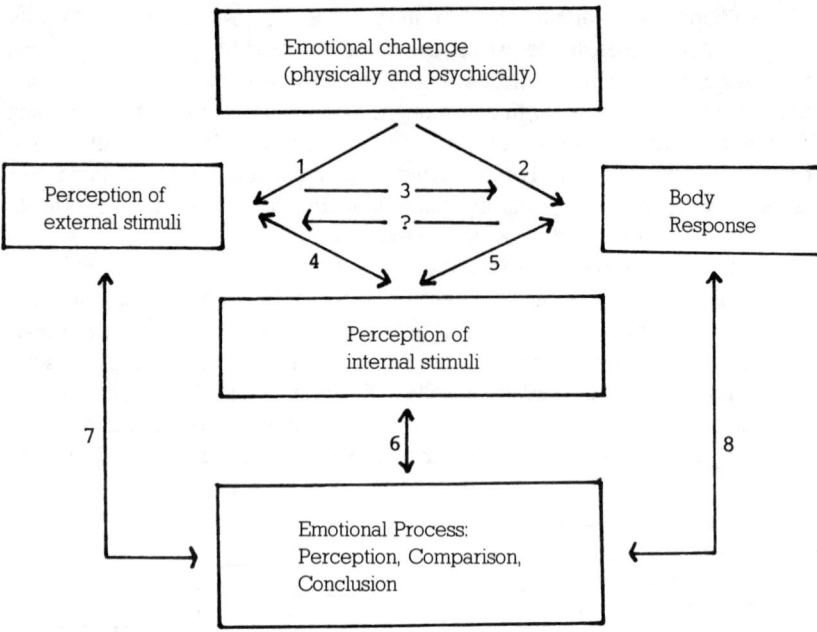

Figure 4. The process of emotional coping.

tems: "The organism that can use symptoms as a source of feedback in order to self-regulate will have a far higher survival rate than the organism that does not perceive and/or use symptom information. Symptoms then, are signals, indicating the current state of the body and/or environment . . ." (Pennebaker, 1982).

Structure of the Interview Guide

The guide consists of 46 pages divided into 15 separately indexed units. This index form makes it possible for the patient to determine the order in which the topics should be discussed. In this manner an unconstrained flow of conversation is achieved.

The interview contains behavior-analytical questions significant to the occurrence of headache, for instance, the questions concerning the course of attack, the localisation of the pain, the releasing stimuli, the resulting circumstances, as well as the medical history of the headaches. Further contents include the social consequences of the disorder, such as the reactions from the immediate environment, the work world, the effect of the headache on patients' general quality of life, family relationships such as those with patients' parents and partner children. Furthermore, we are interested in patients' "self efficacy," that is, the perceived ability of patients to cope with difficult situations. And we are interested in their body perception and their feeling perception, their dealing with stress-prone situations and their spare-time behavior. At the end of the interview, the patients are asked about their expectations concerning therapy and how they assess their prospects for successful treatment. This self-evaluation plays a great role with respect to the question how much the patients can contribute to their own recovery.

The interview lasts between 90 and 150 minutes depending on the conversational activity or passiveness of the patient.

As a conclusion to the interview, the therapist fills out a clinical evaluation form, consisting of 42 judgements. The items refer to the following judgement aspects:

1. Countertransference of the interviewer; these items are to help the therapist remain fair during the judgement process.
2. The patient's style of communication
3. The patient's feeling processes
4. The patient's perception and way of dealing with body functions and processes
5. The patient's possibilities for coping with stress
6. The patient's value system
7. The patient's self-confidence and self-efficacy
8. The patient's expectations concerning therapy
9. The therapy indications for the patient.

The therapist uses an evaluator's manual as an aid in making the evaluation. The manual refers to each of the nine aspects mentioned.

The Initial Interview in Methodological Test

At the University of Ulm the initial interview has so far been tested on more than 150 patients who have come to the Pain Therapy Clinic because of their psychogenic headache. Of those patients, we chose a sample of 35 men and women for quantitative analysis of the qualitative data from the psychodiagnostic evaluation form of the interview guide. Five clinicians observed each of the 35 video-taped interviews and filled out the psychodiagnostic evaluation form for each one. The average reliability of the individual judgements calculated according to the analysis of variance using repeated measurements (Winer, 1962) is 0.79, with a range of 0.44 to 0.93.

Results of the Reliability Study

The most reliable items of the evaluation form refer to

a) the patient's expectations concerning therapy (items 34 to 39)
b) the patient's style of communication (items 7, 8, 9 and 13)
c) the patient's self-efficacy (items 32 and 33)
d) the patient's feeling process (items 14 to 17) and
e) the patient's perception of body functions and processes (items 22 and 25)

Comments

ad a) The interviewer precisely describes and itemizes the existing *possibilities of treatment*. This is precisely commented on by the patients since in general they know very well which therapy form comes nearest to their own expectations, such as acupuncture or medical alternatives to drug treatment.

ad b) The patient's *style of communication* is in some aspects easy to evaluate: The duration of the interview shows whether the patient talks much or little (item 7), whether his or her style of communication is rather reactive or active (item 8), whether the patient accepts the order of the questions in the guide or whether the interviewer is expected to go back and forth in the interview guide. The high intercorrelation between item 9 and item 13, e.g., openness and verbal capacity, is an indication that the inteviewer is regarding the judgement aspects as synonyms and is thus giving way to stereotyped judgements that may be based in his or her social origin, quasi a continental equivalent of the American JAVIS patient type.

ad c) The interviewing questions concerning the patient's *self-efficacy* are strictly adjusted to the corresponding conception of Bandura (1977). Through the patient's answers, the interviewer is able to evaluate precisely the self-efficacy in the evaluation form.

ad d) As to the judgements concerning the patient's *feeling process* there is a high correlation of the items 14 and 16 ("good perception of feelings" and "high power of conception for feelings"): They have been largely used as synonyms. This implication results from the fact that in conversation with the patient, both aspects can only be dealt with verbally. Verbal expression however depends on imaginative faculties. It is typical that item 18 ("inappropriate handling of feelings") is one of the most inadequate items: It contains a hypothetic element which is impossible to register.

Compared with this however, the empirically closely related items 15 and 17, *ability to express feelings* and *readyness to express feelings* can be gathered immediately from the patient's behavior, though the observer is overtaxed when having to differentiate between the aspect of motivation and that of competence as regards the expression of feelings. Therefore, there is a high intercorrelation between these two items, too.

ad e) The most reliable judgements concerning the patient's *body perception process*, item 22 ("strong conception of how to translate physical sensations into verbal form") and item 25 ("relation of physical pain to psychological experiences") are closely correlated. This is in contrast to item 23 ("expression of physical sensation in an inappropriate manner"), which cannot be proved and which belongs to the most unreliable items.

The most unreliable items of the evaluation form refer to two out of four items concerning *stress-coping capacity*. Item 26 ("recognition of stress") and item 27 ("avoidance of stress-prone situations") are also very unreliable although a special theory as to stress-coping capacity has been developed for the interview and, in addition to that, the interview contains patterns of behavior enabling a better judgement of the patient's coping with stress. We assume that the insufficient reliability of the judgements mentioned arises from the discrepancy between the interviewer's impression when analyzing the patterns of behavior and the patient's self-evaluation with respect to his stress-coping capacity. If the evaluation of the interviewer and the self-evaluation of the patient differ too much from one another, the interviewer cannot be sure whether to believe his or her own impression or that of the patient. This reduces the reliability of the evaluation.

Comparison Interviewer-Observer

A Validity Aspect of the Questionnaire

Since the clinicians who observed the video-tapes were the same as those who had conducted the interviews, we were able to calculate criteria of correspondence between the evaluation of the interviewers and their evaluation of the same patient as a video-tape observer up to two months after the interview. This naturally involves a clear change of aspect, so that in addition to a criterion of stability, a partial validation is also involved. The mean correlation of the interviewers with themselves as observers amounted to 0.66.

At the same time we were also able to calculate the correlation of the interviewing clinician's judgment after the discussion, with the judgment of other observers after they had observed the video-tape of the same patient. The mean correlation for this criterion was 0.51.

The Factorial Structure of the Clinical Questionnaire

We carried out a factor analysis of the 42 items of the questionnaire using the mean value of the 5 observers as a data basis taking an N of 35 patients. A factorial structure with 5 factors resulted which explained 69% of the total variance.

Table 1. Results of the r-technique factor analysis based on the 42 items:

5 factors were extracted:

factor	explained variance	extracted % of the variance	% of the variance after rotation
I	37%	53%	44%
II	12%	17%	19%
III	8%	12%	13%
IV	7%	10%	12%
V	5%	8%	11%

Factor I: Requirements for a Patient Suited to Psychotherapy

Table 2. Abridged version of the items – negative and positive values coincide with left and right key.

Factor I:	Loading:	Requirements for a patient suited to psychotherapy
7)	(−0,91)	The patient talks a lot
8)	(+0,90)	Is more active than reactive
9)	(+0,85)	Appears to be open
17)	(−0,85)	Is very ready to show his feelings
22)	(+0,83)	Has a very strong conception of how to translate his physical sensations into verbal form
14)	(+0,83)	Is very aware of his feelings
15)	(−0,83)	Is able to express his feelings very well
16)	(+0,83)	His power of conception of how to handle his feelings verbally is very strong
4)	(+0,82)	I found the patient fascinating
1)	(+0,81)	Experienced the interview as stimulating
19)	(−0,74)	The patient has a strong tendenxy to act out his feelings
20)	(−0,74)	Is easily aroused
11)	(+0,72)	Uses clear concepts when describing psychosociological matters
13)	(−0,68)	Is highly articulate
10)	(−0,68)	I had no difficulties in understanding the patient

The suitability of a patient first is defined by his or her style of communication and emotional experience and second by countertransference aspects of the therapist. In contrast to this concept is the somato-organic orientation of a patient, which makes any psychotherapeutical approach more difficult.

Factor II: Countertransference Aspects of the Interviewers or Observers

Table 3.

Factor II:		**Summary of countertransference aspects**
	Loading:	
5)	(+0,88)	I thought the patient was rather disagreeable
2)	(+0,77)	During the interview I felt ill at ease
23)	(+0,75)	The patient expresses his physical sensations in an inappropriate manner
18)	(+0,72)	Handles through his experience emotionally in an inappropriate manner
12)	(−0,70)	I had difficulties in understanding the patient
31)	(−0,59)	Appears more rigid in respect of his/her convictions
6)	(−0,58)	I feel dissatisfied with the interview

The relationship between patient and clinical observer has failed.

Factor III: Self-Efficacy Aspects of the Patient

Table 4.

Factor III:		**Self-efficacy aspects**
	Loading:	
29)	(+0,87)	The patient resolves stressful situations with difficulty
28)	(+0,72)	Bears stress poorly
26)	(+0,62)	His/her attitude towards further diagnostic medical investigation is positiv
33)	(−0,57)	Has a strong sense of self efficacy

Factor IV: Requirements for Psychosocial Care of the Patient

Table 5.

Factor IV:	Loading:	Requirements for psychosocial care
37)	(−0,79)	The patients attitude to interview based therapy is positive
35)	(+0,59)	Towards alternative therapy forms is positive
39)	(−0,59)	Towards social welfare measure is positive
42)	(+0,58)	Social welfare measure are well suited
30)	(+0,54)	Allows him/herself to be guided by behavior rather than by his/her own needs
40)	(+0,51)	Methods of verbal therapy are very sensible

This factor is determined by the expectations concerning therapy and the question of how and if the patient can be treated, i.e., it stands for the requirements for psychosocial care of the patient. This concept is both defined by the urgency of the expectations concerning therapy and by its suitability for specific interventions.

Factor V: The Requirements for Behavior Therapy Techniques

Table 6.

Factor V:	Loading:	Requirement for behavior therapy techniques
41)	(+0,81)	Methods of behavior therapy are less sensible
32)	(−0,63)	His/her expectation of self efficacy in respect to course of therapy is low

The few high-loading items of this factor stand for a rather unreliable interpretation.

A Patient Typology by a q-Technique Factor Analysis

We then used the body of data to calculate yet a q-technique factor analysis. In this analysis we determined the factor scores for each factor in order to formulate patient types. A factorial structure with 5 factors resulted which explained 73% of the total variance.

Table 7. Results of the q-technique factor analysis based on 35 patients

Factor	total variance	extracted variance	rotated variance	number of patients
I	31%	42%	29%	9
II	18%	25%	28%	9
III	10%	14%	18%	5
IV	8%	10%	13%	4
V	6%	9%	12%	3

Interpretation

Factor I: The So-called "Good Patient"

This type is defined by a clear social adjustment: During the interview i.e., in a situation they are not used to, the patients are accessible and open and always striving for a clear style of communication. They reject social-educational measures. They would indeed make no sense for them, since their problem is not lack of social adjustment but, to the contrary, they are rather likely to be overadaptive. This excessive adjustment could, for instance, prevent them from sup-

Table 8.

Factor I:		The "Good Patient" type
	Loading:	Items with high factor scores:
patient 25	0,85	9) The patient appears reticent
patient 14	0,85	6) I feel satisfied with the interview
patient 35	0,85	
patient 11	0,82	12) I had no difficulties in undstanding the patient
patient 30	0,80	
patient 21	0,76	39) The patient's attitude to social welfare measures is critical
patient 8	0,67	
patient 31	0,62	36) His/her attitude towards further diagnostic medical investigations is critical
patient 22	0,62	
		41) Behavior therapy is very sensible
		42) Social welfare measures are little suited to him/her

plying their own needs. This may explain why the only therapy that seems to be suited for such patients is behavior therapy.

With respect to their attitude toward the therapist, this type of patient reminds one of the typical "good patient" who, with their obligingness, are welcome partners for the observers who thus feel supported in their qualities as therapists and are content with the discussion.

Factor II: The Goal-Oriented Patient

These patients are defined by their well-conceived expectations concerning therapy. They are to be seen as emphatically determined characters having exactly defined ideas about what will be and what will not be of help to them. This concept-oriented behavior accompanies a personality defined more by external norms than by its own needs.

Table 9.

Factor II:		**The goal-oriented patient type**
	Loading:	Items with high factor scores:
patient 28	0,91	15) The patient is not able to express his feelings very well
patient 6	0,96	
patient 10	0,84	35) His/her attitude toward alternative therapy forms is positive
patient 26	0,83	
patient 29	0,80	36) His/her attitude toward further diagnostic investigations is positive
patient 1	0,72	
patient 20	0,70	37) His/her attitude to therapy based on interviews is negative
patient 17	0,64	
patient 23	0,60	38) ... behavior therapy techniques is positive
		39) ... to social welfare measures is negative
		30) The patient allows him/herself to be guided by behavior rather than by external norms
		31) In respect to his/her convictions, the patient appears more rigid
		33) She/he has a strong sense of self-efficacy
		41) Behavior therapy techniques are very sensible
		42) Social welfare measures are not well suited to her/him

This patient type will rather rigidly stick to a persuasion once acquired. In summary, the attributes "action-oriented" and "success-oriented" are the ones that come nearest to what makes the character of this patient type, the more so as such a patients is most distinctly defined by a rather high general self-efficacy.

Because of this high degree of self-efficacy, such patients strive for adoption of all possible forms of therapy that they find suitable. They accept everything: alternative methods as well as further medical-diagnostic investigations as well as behavior therapy. Similar to patient-type I, social welfare measures are of no help to this patient type, since they are characterized less by a lack of social reinforcement, and some kind of social barrier will even stimulate them.

Though this patient-group is primarily defined by its lack of ability to express feelings, their attitude to therapy forms using interview techniques to cope with this deficiency is negative.

This patient type is very similar to the so-called "enlightened patient" (Argelander, 1979). The motivation of these patients is determined by what they know, the degree of their enlightment, and their need for more knowledge. For the most part, such patients have already been working on themselves and use an appropriate vocabulary stemming from the literature, their occupation, or their earlier treatment. They do not play games with their knowledge, but take it seriously, because it is based on strong intellectual needs—it strives for completion, sometimes even for absolute perfection. The highly trained and for the most part very differentiated intellectuality of such patients stands in contrast to the locked-in, stunted emotional life that is very difficult to get at.

At first, patients of this type appear to be the ideal patients—until it turns out that behind their intellectual motility, their real interest, and their convincing conscious motivations, almost insurmountable barriers screen off their emotional life. The barriers are insurmountable because the object relationships that are borne by the emotions are prematurely suppressed and are still bound up with the infantile anxieties that accompany them. So it very often happens that separation anxieties permit the possibilities for satisfaction in the object relationship to retreat for the benefit of admiration for the gleaming intelligence and the documentation of its power.

Factor III: The Alexithymic Patient

Table 10.

Factor III:	Loading:	**The alexithymic patient type** Items with high factor scores:
patient 4	0,74	13) The patient is highly inacrticulate
patient 5	0,66	33) She/he has a very limited sense of self afficacy
patient 16	0,65	37) His/her attitude to interview based on therapy is critical
patient 24	0,60	39) His/her attitude to social welfare measures is critical
		36) ... to further diagnostic medical investigations is critical
		38) ... to behavior therapy techniques is negative

Poor verbal capacity and a rather low general self-efficacy define patient type III as a problematic patient to whom no therapeutic recommendation can be given. Such patients refuse not only medical-diagnostic investigation, but also verbal therapy techniques, just as they will refuse behavior therapy-oriented techniques or social welfare measures. This refusing, failure-oriented attitude is well-suited to producing a therapeutic helplessness on part of the interviewer.

This patient type reminds one of the psychoanalytical character of alexithymia and the unproductive patient (see Argelander, 1979; Haesler, 1979). Analysis of this patient type has, however, not been able to find out whether these patients, characterized as colorless, dull, and reserved are defined as "unproductive" because of a deficiency in their personality structure, or whether they have fallen victim to therapeutic avoidance behavior and, as a result, are often misunderstood (in particular because of their verbal capacity rated as low).

Factor IV: Patient Interested in Psychological Therapy

Table 11.

Factor IV:		**Patient interested in psychological therapy**
	Loading:	Items with high factor scores:
patient 18	0,87	15) The patient is not able to express his feelings very well
patient 12	0,71	
patient 32	0,68	35) His/her attitude to alternative therapy forms is positive
patient 27	0,66	38) . . . to behavior therapy techniques is positive
		40) Methods of verbal therapy are very sensible
		8) The patient is more reactive than active
		36) His/her . . . to further diagnostic medical investigations is critical
		37) His/her . . . to interview based therapy interviews is positive

This patient type is attracted by both, alternative therapy techniques and behavior-therapy techniques, as well as by the adoption of verbal encounters and all introspectively-oriented therapy forms with the same openness, while they refuse any further medical-diagnostic investigation.

Factor V: The Disagreeable Patient

These patients fall into the therapist's disgrace: They are experienced as disagreeable, plaintive, and oversensitive. According to the therapist, these patients work through their experiences in a rather inadequate manner. Compared with the patient types presented above, this patient group is mostly defined by factor scores of countertransference on behalf of the therapist, who cannot find any therapeutic method suited to them. It is possible that this unfavorable constellation is due to the most demanding attitude of the patient group V. They have no

Table 12.

Factor V:		**The disagreeable patient**
	Loading:	Items with high factor scores:
patient 33	0,78	5) The patient was rather disagreeable
patient 19	0,64	18) The patient handles his experiences emotionally in an inappropriate manner
patient 2	0,42	19) She/he has a strong tendency to act out her/his feelings
		24) ... complains about his physical troubles very much
		35) The patient's attitude towards further diagnostic medical investigations is positive
		39) ... to social welfare measures is positive

confidence in the findings recorded so far and feel uneasy about them, so they demand further medical-diagnostic investigation and, in addition, plead for social welfare measures, which have to be provided as practical as can be and without any delay.

This patient type reminds one of the "demanding patient" described by Argelander (1979):

"Often he already has a number of attempts at treatment behind him. Thus, for example, he would like to have an elderly, especially experienced, and gentle interviewer. Such high demand is in contrast to a lack of... That is also why he is quickly offended or disappointed, feels that he is being misunderstood, and sometimes complains. For the most part it is only at this point that the actual poverty of this real existence, which is hidden behind his excessive demands, is divulged. This discrepancy between his demanding behavior and his personal possibilities is the criterion for this type of patient. Behind this behavior are concealed persons with disturbed relations to reality, who, despite their great demands, actually lead a miserable existence. In the conversation situation they are unreliable and uncontrollable, and for the most part arouse reactions of pity, which spoil a correct evaluation of them. Not seldom, this type exhibits psychopathic traits. In this case, they commit large or small acts of tactlessness and provoke a hidden or an open rejection. The patient has an unfavorable effect on the interviewer." (Argelander, 1979).

Conclusion

The results of the data analysis presented above prove that the interview guide, despite its qualitative acquisition mode, leads to quantitative clinical evaluations that are reliable, satisfactorily stable, and sufficiently valid with respect to interviewer and observer. The conditions for our investigation were:

1. Intensive training of the interviewers conducting the initial interviews for psychodiagnostic clarification.
2. The observers as well had to go through an intensive training.

In addition to a general introduction of how to enter and carry on a conversation, the training program of the interviewer also comprises the aspects of the headache event that are important for behavioral medicine.

The observers were instructed by means of the video-taped initial interviews. As an aid in making evaluation of the 42 judgements on the clinical evaluation form, we have designed a manual.

References

Argelander, H. (1979). *The initial interview in psychotherapy*. New York: Human Sciences Press.

Bakal, D.A. (1982). *The psychobiology of chronic headache*. New York: Springer-Verlag.

Bandura, A. (1977). Self-efficacy: Toward a unifying theory of behavioral change. *Psychological Review, 84,* 191—215.

Bischoff, C., Zenz, H., & Traue, H. (1986). Primärer Kopfschmerz. In T. v. Uexküll (Ed.), *Psychosomatische Medizin* (pp. 565—576). München: Urban & Schwarzenberg.

Cronbach, L., & Gleser, G.C. (1957). *Psychological tests and personnel decisions*. Urbana: University of Illinois Press.

Friedman, A.P. (1962). Ad hoc committee on classification of headache. *J. Amer. Med. Assoc., 179,* 717—718.

Gerber, W.D., & Haag, G. (1982). *Migräne*. Berlin: Springer-Verlag.

Guilford J.P. (1965). *Persönlichkeit*. Weinheim: Beltz.

Haesler, L. (1979). Zur Technik des Interviews bei "unergiebigen" Patienten. *Psyche, 19,* 157—182.

Matarazzo, J.D. (1965). The interview. In B.B. Wolmann (Ed.), *Handbook of clinical psychology*. New York: McGraw-Hill.

Pennebaker, J.W. (1982). *The psychology of physical symptom*. New York: Springer-Verlag.

Philips, C. (1980). Recent developments in tension headache research: Implication for understanding and management of the disorder. In S. Rachman (Ed.), *Contributions to medical psychology, Vol. 2* (pp. 113—130). Oxford: Pergamon Press.

Winer, B.J. (1962). *Statistical principles in experimental design*. New York: McGraw-Hill.

Zuckerman, M., Kolin, E.A., Price, L., & Zoob, I. (1964). Development of a sensation seeking scale. *J. Consult., 28,* 477—482.

APPENDIX

Headache Interview

Date: ....

Patient's name: ....

....

Date of birth: ....

....

Address: ....

....

Telephone: ....

Interviewer: ....

Copyright (c) by H. Zenz & G. Manok, Ulm

Course of Attack

What seems to be the trouble?
(Metaphors! Feelings! Emotions! Phantasies!)

Can you *describe* a typical headache attack?

How strong are the headaches?
(not in figures!)

How long does the attack last as a rule?

How do you *feel* during an attack?

What *thoughts* go through your head when you experience this pain?

Have you ever noticed that your mood changes during the pain? In what way does it change?

How do you behave during an attack? For example, do you try to reduce the worst pain with medicine, or do you go and lie down?

Localisation

Where do you have the headache?
(verbalization! phantasies!)

Frequency, Time, Trigger

How often on average during the week/month do you suffer from headaches at present?

Do the headaches occur on certain days, for example weekends or holidays?

Have you ever considered *why* you *react* with headaches at certain times, but are free of symptoms on other days? (If necessary give examples.)

Can you *picture* a situation in which you would promptly react with a headache? Have you *noticed changes in yourself* already hours or days before the onset of pain which lead you to expect an imminent attack? If so, were you perhaps in a bad mood, or, on the contrary, a particularly good mood?

Are there *phases* in which you are not pestered by your headaches?

Chronicle of Headaches

How long have you suffered headaches?

Can you still *remember the situations* in which you were first aware of headaches?

Which feelings did these situations release and how did you feel at that moment?

Earlier headache episodes:

Did you have headaches earlier from time to time?

If this is the case, in which *situations* did these pains arise?

What *did you do* to stop the headaches?

Social Consequences and Reactions of Social Environment

What is the attitude of the *members of your family* to you illness?

Are they *understanding*?

How do members of your family react when you have a headache?

Is there someone else in your *family* who suffers chronically like you? In other words do you have a companion in suffering?

How do you *feel* when you have a headache? Do you feel *uncomfortable* when you have to *depend on the consideration of other people*? Can you describe your thoughts and feelings that come to mind in these circumstances?

Has anything *changed* in your *family* since your headaches have arisen?

How do your *friends* and *acquaintances* behave in relation to your affliction?

Has anything *changed* in *relation* to your friends and acquaintances since then?

What are your experiences with *doctors* whom you have asked for help?

Did you feel *understood* to a degree by them, or did you have the feeling that your affliction was *not taken seriously*?

Have you sought alternative help as well? I am thinking of homeopaths for example . . .

If this is the case, what are your *experiences with alternative medicine*?

And what do you yourself think of your headaches? *Do you believe that you are ill*?

Motivation for visiting the doctor:

Now you have certainly been battling with your headaches for a long time. *Why* have you actually gone *to the doctor just now*?

Place of Work

Now would you please describe the nature of your work to me?

Does headache hinder your *work*? How does it make itself felt?

What do your *colleagues/superiors* do when you have a headache?

Can you describe the *thoughts* and *feelings* that go through your head at such reactions?

Do your colleagues act differently toward you since you have suffered from headaches?

Could you imagine yourself *taking sick-leave* at the moment of worst pain?

Are you afraid that you could *lose your job* if you show that you suffer from headaches?

How would you describe your *relationship* with your *colleagues*?

How do your *colleagues* see you?

And how would you *describe yourself*?

Can you *express* yourself in your job about as much as you would like?

Do you repeatedly come across *situations* where you wish you would at *long last change*?

Are you *contented* with your job/your work as a housewife?

What *significance* do you attribute to your *job*? Do you think your job is a necessary evil, or do you value some aspects of your work?

Are you doing the kind of *work* you always wanted to do?

If not, why were you not able to fulfill your original wishes concerning work?

How do you feel now about the work you have chosen?

Do you sometimes toy with the idea to *get away* from the *tedious daily routine*, to emigrate to Australia, to keep sheep, or to retrain for a new job?

Unemployment

How long have you been unemployed?

How do you *cope with unemployment*? Can you describe the worst difficulties?

Is there something you especially *miss* at the moment?

How do you pass the time?

How does your *family/partner* feel about your unemployment? Does the fact that you are without a job sometimes cause *arguments*?

Please, imagine, you have found a *new job*. How would *things be different*?

Why does the fact that you are unemployed stop you from doing these things now?

Quality of Life

Can you try and think back to when you were not yet troubled so badly by your headaches. What *has changed since then*? Is there something particularly lacking in your life from that time?

How much do you feel your *zest for life has been curtailed*?

Why do you allow your headaches to become such a handicap to you?

Now just imagine your pains would disappear from one day to the next. How would that change your life?

Has your temperament changed at all during the course of your ailment?

Would you say you are satisfied with yourself, your achievements until now and your private life generally? Or, do you tend to be dissatisfied with your lot?

Singles

What do you *do* after *work*? How do you spend your *weekends*?

Would you say you *find it easy* to make *contacts*? *How important* is *human contact* for you?

Do you *find it difficult* to live *alone*?

Don't you sometimes feel lonely?

Did you have a relationship in former times?

Were you happy then?

Why did this *relationship end*? Are you still *sad* about the separation, or are you on the contrary quite *pleased* about it?

Are you afraid of a future on your own?

What do you do when things *get on top of you*?

Why do you think you are living on *your own*? Would you like to share your life with a partner?

Former relationships:

What characteristics did you especially value in your *former partner*?

What do you *miss* most being on *your own*?

How do you manage your *sexuality*?

Are you *optimistic* that one day you will *find a partner* who is compatible with you, or do you feel continually *accident prone* when it comes to love?

Family

How would you describe your *relationship* with your *family*, also in emotional terms?

And how do your *relatives see you*?

Do you wish your *relatives saw you differently*?

Do *problems* in your *family* always have the *same cause*?

In what way do you try to resolve the *problems* in your family?

Who *determines what happens* in your family? Who signs the contracts, or school reports? Who decides were you go on vacation, what car to buy, and which school the children go to?

Would you describe your family life as *harmonious*, or are there things that you continually clash over?

Could you please describe in your *imagination* what an *ideal family* would be like?

Have your *expectations* in this respect been *fulfilled* so far? Or, is there something lacking in your family life that stops you from feeling happy?

Relationship with Partner

What do you feel about your *relationship* with your husband/partner/wife/girlfriend?

Do you have the impression that your *partner* is the kind of person who is *sensitive* to the needs of others?

Do you feel *secure with your partner* when you are *feeling unwell* and you need to be cared for and comforted?

What is your *husband's/wife's occupation*?

Do you feel that the *wishes and expectations* that you had at the beginning of the relationship are *fulfilled* in the way you and your partner relate? Or, do you think that your feelings are ignored, and that too *little considertion* is given to your ideas, thoughts and moods?

What has your husband/partner, wife/girlfriend got to *offer* you *emotionally*?

And what have *you* got to *offer emotionally* to your husband/partner/wife/girlfriend?

Is there anything in the *relationship* with your husband/partner/wife/girlfriend that worries you?

Are you sometimes *jealous* of your partner? Do you have reason to be jealous? And what about your partner? Does she/he ever feel *jealous* about you?

Sexuality

Is it alright with you if we now talk about the sexual content of your relationship?

What do you feel about your sexual relationship with your husband/partner, wife/girlfriend? Do you think that what you *experience sexually* together is important for your *relationship*?

Do you *enjoy* being *affectionate* to your husband/partner/wife/girlfriend?

Do you *enjoy lovemaking*?

How *often* and *when do you make love*? Do you sometimes wish you would make love more often? Or, would you actually prefer it if it happened less often?

Would you say your sexual life was *fulfilling* with regard to your *own wishes* and *expectations*, or do you long for your partner to be more giving?

If you think the latter is true, why is it that *you don't receive enough*, do you think?

Do you have the impression that your relationship is clouded by *sexual tensions*?

Are you actually *happy* in your marriage/relationship?

Self-Effectiveness ("Efficacy")

Do you think it is fair to say that you succeed at everything you attempt? Or, do you often say to yourself: I'll *never manage* that.

How do you *deal with problems* when you are *not* exactly *sure* whether you will be able to resolve them? Do you feel intimidated by such situations, or do you *feel confident to tackle them*?

(Ask for examples!)

Have you often experienced *failure* in the *past*? Can you think of an *example*?

Do you normally perceive solutions to *problems* to be *more difficult* to achieve than they really are?

Do you think you *take it well* when you have *been unsuccessful* or does your self-confidence completely collapse in these situations?

Are you able to *relish* your assertiveness when it has allowed you to be *successful* in a *difficult situation*?

What does *success mean* to you?

Are there *models* from the past that guided you with regard to your behavior and feelings?

Sporting Activities—Attitude Toward Own Body:

How do you keep fit?

Do you have enough *opportunity* besides your occupation/housework to keep *physically active*?

Do you feel that this *compensation is good for you*?

If you don't actively engage in a sport: Do you feel you *need a compensation* like sport?

Physical and Emotional Perception

Do you often *find* that you are under *stress*? Can you describe a few *situations* when this happens?

Do you get a kick out of *stressful situations* or do you try to *avoid* them as much as possible?

Probes into behavior:

Directions for the therapist:

Please try to match the behavior probes with the real life situation of the patient! You might find the information gathered hitherto helpful, especially the comments of the patient under the heading of "self-effectiveness."

Please imagine you are in a *terrible rush:* The phone rings non-stop just as you are about to rush your children to the nursery and your train is leaving in 20 minutes . . .

What *feelings* and *thoughts* come spontaneously to mind?

Do you actually *notice* when *you* are *under stress*?

Please imagine you have *made a mistake:* For days now you have been sick of your work. You are in a dreadful mood, dissatisfied and irritable. This morning your work is taking your forever. You make a major blunder because you lost your concentration. Suddenly, your boss appears behind you.

Painful situations:

Imagine your boss accuses you of carelessness! But actually the thing had nothing to do with you and you say so to your superior, but unexpectedly your colleague supports your boss. What *thoughts* and *feelings* spontaneously come to your mind?

What do you actually *feel* when somebody *hurts* or *offends* you?

How do you *deal* with such a *stress situation*? Are you able to tolerate it, or do you find it difficult to take?

What do you do to *manouvre yourself out* of such a situation?

What do you do in a *situation* that *threatens to get on top of you*? Do you manage to pause and take a deep breath to ease the tension or do you get into a state?

One person gets clammy hands because of sheer nervous tension, another's heart is in their mouth when they are frightened. Do you also react *physically* when you are in an *emotional state*?

Do you believe that you also express these sensations bodily?

Do you *dare to show* other people how you are feeling?

If not, why not? What reactions are you *afraid* of?

How do you manage best to *relax physically*? I am thinking here of an afernoon nap, a visit to a sauna or the swimming pool . . .

Attitude Toward Leisure Activities

What do you most look forward to *after work*?

How do you spend the major part of your free time?

There are a variety of leisure activities, TV, knitting, painting, writing, sport, dancing, going to the pub, listening to music, clubs, cooking, reading . . .

Which is your *favorite hobby*?

Enquire about: handcrafts, intellectual or physical activities. Entertainment. Education. Political/religious/community activities. Do you participate in . . .

How much free time do you allocate to the *family* in the arrangement of your working hours and in the making of plans for the future?

Do you think that these *interests enrich* your life?

Do these *hobbies* (and your involvement in other activties) help you to *manage* your *headaches*?

Quite *apart* from these is there something else you *would like to do* in your free time?

Why then don't you do it?

Do you occasionally see your *friends* and *acquaintances*?

Where and at what occasion do you see them?

Is it important for you to *discuss* with your friends and acquaintances the kind of *problems* you cannot discuss at all, or not as fully as you would like, with your family?

Could you *do without* the contact with your friends?

Which aspects of these friendships are particularly important to you?

Expectations of Treatment and Receptiveness Toward Treatment

Do you *yourself* have any *idea* how we could help you to deal with these headaches?

Directions for the therapist:

Carefully describe all the *different possibilities* to the patient:

1. Explanation of all the *physiological* interventions (acupuncture, massage, heat treatment, health farms)
Do you believe that we could help you with any of those?
Do you have any *further questions* concerning this?

2. Explanation of all *other medical forms of intervention* (medication, homeopathic treatment, etc.)
Do you believe that we could help you with any of these?
Have you got any *questions about this*?

3. Explanation of a *competence training for psychic deficiencies* (self-awareness training, aggression-management training, stress awareness and management, self-assertiveness training, relaxation exercises).
Do you believe that we might be able to help with any of those?
Have you got any more questions about this?

4. Description of the *psychotherapeutic* approach:
Do you believe that . . .
Have you any more *questions about this*?

5. Description of *health* and *fitness training*:
Do you believe that . . .
Have you any more *questions about this*?

6. Description of the *social welfare support system* (introduction to a counselor educational welfare officer, help with the search for a new work place, etc.)
Do you believe that . . .
Do you have any *questions about this*?

Or would you prefer if we investigated the causes of your headaches more intensively and *continued with the diagnosis*?

Possibilities of Self-Cure

Do you believe that you yourself could *contribute* to *overcome* these headaches?

If you fight with all the means in your power to get rid of these headaches, how *probable* do you think it is that you *will achieve* your aim?

How would that improve your situation?

And if you *don't succeed* in getting rid of your headaches—what would that mean for you?

Let us imagine that *our* efforts are unable to change your headaches. What will you do next?

Psychodiagnostic Evaluation of the Interview

Patient: . . . .

Date: . . . .

Interviewer: . . . .

. . . .

1. I experienced the interview as
   rather tiring—3 2 1 0 1 2 3—rather stimulating.

2. During the interview I felt
   at ease—3 2 1 0 1 2 3—ill at ease.

3. During the interview I felt
   rather superior—3 2 1 0 1 2 3—rather inferior.

4. I found the patient
   rather boring—3 2 1 0 1 2 3—very fascinating.

5. I thought the patient was
   rather agreeable—3 2 1 0 1 2 3—rather disagreeable.

6. I feel
   dissatisfied—3 2 1 0 1 2 3—satisfied
   with the interview.

7. The patient talks a
   lot—3 2 1 0 1 2 3—very little.

8. During the interview the patient is
   more reactive—3 2 1 0 1 2 3—than active.

9. During the interview the patient appeared to
   be reticent—3 2 1 0 1 2 3—open.

10. It was
    easy—3 2 1 0 1 2 3—difficult
    for me to form a picture of the patient in my mind.

11. When describing psycho/sociological matters the patient uses
    vague—3 2 1 0 1 2 3—clear concepts.

12. I had
    difficulties—3 2 1 0 1 2 3—no difficulties
    in understanding the patient.

13. The patient is
    highly articulate—3 2 1 0 1 2 3—inarticulate.

14. The patient is
    hardly aware—3 2 1 0 1 2 3—very aware
    of his/her feelings.

15. The patient is able to express his/her feelings
    very well—3 2 1 0 1 2 3—very poorly.

16. The patient's power of conception of how to handle his/her feelings verbally is
    very limited—3 2 1 0 1 2 3—very strong.

17. The patient is
    very ready—3 2 1 0 1 2 3—less ready
    to show his/her feelings during the interview.

18. The patient handles through his/her experiences emotionally in an
    appropriate—3 2 1 0 1 2 3—inappropriate
    manner.

19. The patient has
    a strong tendency—3 2 1 0 1 2 3—a weak tendency
    to act out his/her feelings.

20. The patient is
    easily—3 2 1 0 1 2 3—less easily
    aroused.

21. The patient is able to perceive his/her physical sensations
    very well—3 2 1 0 1 2 3—very badly.

22. The patient has a
    very poor—3 2 1 0 1 2 3—very strong
    conception of how to translate his/her physical sensations into verbal form.

23. The patient expresses his physical sensations in an
    appropriate—3 2 1 0 1 2 3—inappropriate
    manner.

24. The patient complains about his/her physical troubles
    very much—3 2 1 0 1 2 3—very little.

25. The patient can relate his/her physical pains to his/her psychological experiences
    very well—3 2 1 0 1 2 3—very poorly.

26. The patient can recognize and assess his/her stress
    very poorly—3 2 1 0 1 2 3—very well.

27. The patient is able to avoid situations of stress
    very well—3 2 1 0 1 2 3—very poorly.

28. The patient bears stress
    poorly—3 2 1 0 1 2 3—well.

29. The patient resolves stressful situations
    with difficulty—3 2 1 0 1 2 3—with ease.

30. The patient allows him/herself to be guided by behavior rather than
    by external norms—3 2 1 0 1 2 3—by his/her own needs.

31. With respect to his/her convictions, the patient appears
    more rigid—3 2 1 0 1 2 3—more flexible.

32. The patient's expectation of self-efficacy with respect to the course of therapy is
    low—3 2 1 0 1 2 3—high.

33. The patient has
    a very limited sense of self-efficacy—3 2 1 0 1 2 3—a strong sense of self-efficacy.

34. The patient's attitude to medical school therapy courses is
    positive—3 2 1 0 1 2 3—negative.

35. The patient's attitude toward alternative therapy forms is
    critical—3 2 1 0 1 2 3—positive.

36. The patient's attitude toward further diagnostic medical investigations is
    critical—3 2 1 0 1 2 3—positive.

37. The patient's attitude toward therapy based on interviews is
    positive—3 2 1 0 1 2 3—negative.

38. The patient's attitude toward behavior therapy techniques is
    negative—3 2 1 0 1 2 3—positive.

39. The patient's attitude toward social welfare measures is
    positive—3 2 1 0 1 2 3—critical.

40. I find methods of verbal therapy
    less sensible—3 2 1 0 1 2 3—very sensible.

41. I find behavior therapy
    very sensible—3 2 1 0 1 2 3—less sensible.

42. I find social welfare measures
    not well suited—3 2 1 0 1 2 3—well suited to him/her.

The German Version of the McGill Pain Questionnaire: The Münchner Schmerzwortskala

Gabriela Mendl* and Christoph Stein**

This study presents a German version of the *McGill Pain Questionnaire* (MPQ) developed by strict adherence to the methodology originally employed by Melzack and Torgerson. Three groups of subjects participated in our study: The first group (n=40) was used to construct a 5-point intensity scale; the second group (n=42) was presented a preliminary translation of the MPQ and asked to assign an intensity rating out of the 5-point intensity scale to each of the 78 adjectives; in the last phase, adjectives whose mean ratings differed markedly from those in the original MPQ were resubmitted, along with 3—4 synonyms to a third group (n=40), which was again asked to assign an intensity value to each word. Finally, the adjectives whose ratings best corresponded, and thus resulted in congruent rank positions, to those of the English originals were selected. The present counterpart to the MPQ retains the original grouping of adjectives, the identical number of words per group as well as their rank positions within groups. Thus, a comparison between German and English mean ratings rank values and number of words chosen as well as statistical calculations derived therefrom is feasible.

Among the various verbal methods of pain measurement, the *McGill Pain Questionnaire* (MPQ) represents one of the most widely used tools for assessment of clinical pain. Since it was developed by Melzack in 1975, it has been used in more than 70 studies.

The verbal method of pain measurement is based on the asumption made by Melzack and Torgerson (1971) that the experience of pain has a multidimensional character. They conceptualized pain as a three-dimensional experience: sensory-discriminative, motivational-affective, and cognitive-evaluative. Factorial studies on low back pain patients (McCreary, Turner, & Dawson, 1981; Prieto et al., 1980) supported this conceptional model.

The *McGill Pain Questionnaire* consists primarily of three major categories of word descriptors that are used by patients to specify subjective pain experi-

---

*Institute of Medical Psychology, Ludwig-Maximilians-University, Munich, FRG
**Institute of Anesthesiology, Ludwig-Maximilians-University, Munich, FRG
The authors wish to thank Heike Schneider, Inge Fottner, Sigrid Schiffelholz, Hildegard Neubrand, Dr. Hans-Jörg Ebell, Toni Shippenberg, and Dietmar Heel for their invaluable assistance and stimulating discussions.

ence. The classes are: First, words that describe *sensory qualities* in terms of temporal, spatial, pressure, thermal, and other properties; second, words that describe *affective qualities* in terms of tension, fear, and autonomic properties; and third, *evaluative words* that describe the subjective overall intensity of the total experience of pain. The categories comprise a total list of 78 words, which are grouped into 20 subclasses arranged in increasing order of pain intensity within each subclass. Each descriptor has one rank and one scale value obtained by testing groups of patients, physicians, and medical students. In the first part of the original study, subjects were asked to classify words obtained from clinical literature relating to pain into smaller groups that described different aspects of pain experience. The second part was an attempt to determine the pain intensities implied by the words within each subclass. Therefore, lists of words were presented to subjects who were asked to assign an intensity value to each word, using a five-point numerical scale ranging from least pain to worst pain. The data were analyzed to provide a mean rating and standard deviation for each word. The rank position occupied by words within subclasses was then determined on the basis of their mean ratings.

The following indices are derived from the questionnaire (Melzack & Torgerson, 1971): (1) the pain rating index (PRI(S)), based on two types of numerical values that can be assigned to each word descriptor; (2) the present pain intensity index (PPI); and (3) an additional measure related to pain intensity designated as the total number of words chosen (NWC).

Experience has shown the high degree of agreement on the intensity relationships among pain descriptors by patients who had different cultural, socioeconomic, and educational backgrounds in different English-speaking countries (Melzack, 1983).

In the meantime, the *McGill Pain Questionnaire* has been translated into other languages. Besides unpublished Swedish and Hungarian versions, there are adaptions in French (cit. Lahuerta, Smith, & Martinez-Lage, 1982), Spanish (Lahuerta, Smith, & Martinez-Lage, 1982), Finnish (Ketovuori & Pöntinen, 1981), Italian (Maiani & Sanavio, 1985), Chinese (Chen & Hui, 1984), Arabic (Harrison, 1988) and German (Kiss, Müller, & Abel, 1987; Radvila et al., 1987). Since, however, the existing German translations by Kiss et al. (1987) and Radvila et al. (1987) were not developed in a manner similar to the original version, direct comparisons of ratings, rank positions, and statistical calculations to those of the original version are precluded.

Thus, the aim of our study was to develop a German version of the *McGill Pain Questionnaire* (Stein et al., 1987; Stein & Mendl, 1988) employing a methodology as similar as possible to the one used by Melzack and Torgerson (1971).

Methods and Results

We used 122 normal subjects of different levels of education, excluding physicians, other health care related personnel, or patients suffering from chronic pain.

Experiment I

A first group of 40 sucjects was used for the definition of 5 anchor words of the intensity scale. The subjects were 13 males and 27 females, aged between 21–79 years. Each subject was shown a lit of 6 adjectives concerning pain intensity. They were then asked to mark the position of each adjective on a 10-cm visual analogue scale (Huskisson, 1985) bearing at the ends the adjectives "gerade wahrnehmbar" (barely noticeable) and "unerträglich" (unbearable).

The mean scale values of the following three adjectives were approximately equidistant and showed relatively low standard deviation values: "mäßig" (moderate) (mean = 2.4), "mittel" (median) (mean = 4.3), "stark" (intense) (mean = 7.3). Thus, a five-point intensity scale consisting of the following was derived: "gerade wahrnehmbar, mäßig, mittel, stark, unerträglich."

Experiment II

The 78 descriptors of the MPQ were translated into German with the assistance of language teachers, philologists, psychologists, physicians, and laypersons. The second group of 42 subjects, 21 males and 21 females, aged between 22–76 years, was then asked to assign an intensity rating (1–5) out of the foregoing intensity scale to each of the 78 adjectives. The mean ratings of descriptors were then compared to those of the original version (Melzack & Torgerson, 1971).

Experiment III

Fourteen descriptors whose mean ratings differed markedly from those of the original version were resubmitted, along with three to four synonyms to a third group of 40 subjects, 26 females and 14 males, aged between 21–79 years. They were again asked to assign an intensity rating ranging from 1–5 out of the intensity scale to each of the descriptors. Finally, the adjectives whose ratings best corresponded, and thus resulted in congruent rank positions, to those of the English originals were selected. The mean ratings (mean) and standard deviations (SD) of descriptors obtained by the German-speaking subjects and by the English-speaking patients (Melzack & Torgerson, 1971) are reported in Table 1.

The present questionnaire retains the original grouping of adjectives, the identical number of words per group as well as their rank positions within groups.

Table 1. Classes of pain descriptors (in English and German languages) as rated by English-speaking patients and by German normal subjects.

Classes	Descriptors	English		Descriptors	German	
		Mean	SD		Mean	SD
1. Temporal	flickering	1.89	0.94	flatternd	1.75	0.93
	quivering	2.50	0.83	zitternd	2.03	0.95
	pulsing	2.56	0.92	pulsierend	2.75	0.74
	throbbing	2.68	1.00	pochend	3.43	0.78
	beating	2.70	0.98	schlagend	3.83	0.78
	pounding	2.85	1.14	hämmernd	4.15	0.86
2. Spatial	jumping	2.60	0.75	sprunghaft	2.73	0.88
	flashing	2.75	0.97	einschießend	3.58	0.96
	shooting	3.42	0.90	blitzartig	3.68	0.76
3. Punctuate pressure	pricking	1.94	1.11	pieksend	1.65	0.77
	boring	2.05	0.83	bohrend	3.25	0.95
	drilling	2.75	1.37	aufbohrend	4.00	0.73
	stabbing	3.45	0.89	erstechend	4.42	0.63
	lancinating	3.50	0.98	niederstechend	4.50	0.55
4. Incisive pressure	sharp	2.95	0.94	scharf	3.40	0.71
	cutting	3.20	0.95	schneidend	3.73	0.64
	lacerating	3.64	1.16	zerreissend	4.58	0.64
5. Constrictive pressure	pinching	1.95	0.82	zwickend	1.90	0.81
	pressing	2.42	0.90	drückend	2.40	0.74
	gnawing	2.53	0.77	nagend	3.00	0.75
	cramping	2.75	0.79	krampfend	3.70	0.62
	crushing	3.58	1.02	erdrückend	4.30	0.69

Table 1. (continued)

Classes	Descriptors	English Mean	SD	Descriptors	German Mean	SD
6. Traction pressure	tugging	2.16	0.60	ziehend	2.33	0.57
	pulling	2.35	0.59	zerrend	2.98	0.70
	wrenching	3.47	0.90	reißend	3.60	0.71
7. Thermal	hot	2.47	0.85	heiß	3.10	0.74
	burning	2.95	0.85	brennend	3.58	0.68
	scalding	3.50	0.98	glühend	4.18	0.81
	searing	3.88	0.89	siedend	4.63	0.71
8. Brightness	tingling	1.60	0.68	kribbelnd	1.30	0.49
	itchy	1.70	0.80	juckend	1.73	0.64
	smarting	2.00	0.82	beißend	2.85	0.74
	stinging	2.25	0.85	stechend	3.45	0.90
9. Dullness	dull	1.60	0.68	dumpf	2.35	0.62
	sore	1.90	0.64	wund	2.50	0.75
	hurting	2.45	1.14	weh	2.78	1.00
	aching	2.50	1.28	schmerzend	3.05	0.82
	heavy	2.95	0.94	heftig	3.98	0.53
10. Sensory: Miscellaneous	tender	1.35	0.59	weich	1.33	0.62
	taut	2.36	1.01	angespannt	2.20	0.70
	rasping	2.61	0.92	kratzend	2.20	0.77
	splitting	3.10	1.21	spaltend	3.38	0.81
11. Tension	tiring	2.42	0.69	ermüdend	2.33	0.80
	exhausting	2.63	0.96	erschöpfend	3.23	0.83

Table 1. (continued)

Classes	Descriptors	English		Descriptors	German	
		Mean	SD		Mean	SD
12. Autonomic	sickening	2.75	0.79	ekelhaft	2.55	0.80
	suffocating	3.45	1.14	erstickend	4.30	0.67
13. Fear	fearful	3.30	0.92	bedrohlich	3.95	0.68
	frightful	3.53	0.77	schrecklich	4.23	0.66
	terrifying	3.95	1.08	entsetzlich	4.65	0.48
14. Punishment	punishing	3.50	0.79	plagend	3.23	0.53
	gruelling	3.73	0.80	strafend	3.50	0.72
	cruel	3.95	0.89	gemein	3.75	0.71
	vicious	4.26	0.99	bösartig	4.13	0.65
	killing	4.50	0.61	mörderisch	4.88	0.34
15. Affective-evaluative-sensory Miscellaneous	wretched	3.16	0.83	elend	3.50	0.96
	blinding	3.45	1.00	erblindend	4.33	0.87
16. Evaluative	annoying	1.89	0.76	störend	2.38	0.67
	troublesome	2.42	0.69	ärgerlich	2.45	0.60
	miserable	2.85	0.96	erbärmlich	3.76	0.48
	intense	3.75	1.12	intensiv	4.08	0.66
	unbearable	4.42	1.07	unerträglich	4.93	0.47
17. Sensory: Miscellaneous	spreading	3.30	0.98	sich ausbreitend	2.83	0.84
	radiating	3.38	1.15	ausstrahlend	3.03	0.77
	penetrating	3.72	0.89	eindringend	3.40	0.74
	piercing	3.78	0.58	durchdringend	4.23	0.70

Table 1. (continued)

Classes	Descriptors	English		Descriptors	German	
		Mean	SD		Mean	SD
18. Sensory: Miscellaneous	tight	2.25	0.91	straff	2.33	0.73
	numbing	2.10	0.88	taub	2.35	1.08
	drawing	2.53	0.84	zusammenziehend	3.03	0.73
	squeezing	2.35	0.81	quetschend	3.83	0.64
	tearing	3.68	0.93	zerreißend	4.40	0.63
19. Sensory	cool	/	/	kühl	1.75	0.59
	cold	/	/	kalt	2.53	0.78
	freezing	/	/	eisig	3.53	0.91
20. Affective-evaluative: Miscellaneous	nagging	2.25	0.79	hartnäckig	3.18	0.75
	nauseating	2.74	0.93	übelerregend	4.03	0.62
	agonizing	3.20	1.67	quälend	4.15	0.43
	dreadful	4.11	0.76	furchtbar	4.20	0.65
	torturing	4.53	0.70	marternd	4.73	0.45

Discussion

The aim of this study was to develop a German semantic key as close as possible to the English original. In view of cross-cultural investigations, we decided to preserve the subdivision of words into classes and subclasses in order to enable a direct comparison of mean ratings and rank positions of descriptors to those of the original version. In contrast to the original study using physicians, patients, and students (Melzack & Torgerson, 1971), we chose a more heterogeneous group of normal subjects, whose responses were not biased by professional acquaintance of the subject or personal experience with chronic pain syndromes.

Our study differs from the aforementioned German adaptations (Kiss, Müller, & Abel, 1987; Radvila et al., 1987) in the following points:

Kiss, Müller, and Abel (1987) provided a word-by-word translation of the MPQ which sought to rate relative intensities within each subclass. This thesis, however, was not tested in subjects. In our study, each descriptor's intensity value was obtained on a five-point intensity scale and rank positions of descriptors were established accordingly. Moreover, they used only one specific group of subjects, namely, cancer pain patients. Thus the choice of descriptors was biased by a specific experience of pain. The present study, by employing a heterogeneous group of subjects, provides a non-biased list of adjectives which is applicable for multiple types of pain. Recently, Radvila et al. (1987) developed another German adaptation of the MPQ, which, however, consists of a set of only 51 adjectives assigned to 17 groups of three each, thus precluding a direct comparison of ratings and rank positions with those obtained by the original.

The present version permits the calculation of mean scale values, rank values, and the number of words chosen (NWC) in a fashion identical to the original one (Melzack & Torgerson, 1971). The pain rating index based on meanscale values, PRI(S), as well as that based on rank values, PRI(R), can be derived accordingly. Because of our rigorous adherence to the original methodology, these values can be directly compared with values obatined by the English version.

The original MPQ has been subjected to a variety of experimental studies trying to evaluate the psychometric standards, such as reliability, validity, and objectivity of the MPQ in human pain assessment (Bradley et al., 1981; Gracely, McGrath, & Dubner, 1978; Kremer & Atkinson, 1981).

Recent findings (Prieto & Geisinger, 1983) provide relatively strong support for the questionnaire's three-dimensional structure, which has been replicated in both clinical (Byrne et al., 1982; Prieto & Geisinger, 1983; Reading, 1979) and laboratory settings (Crockett, Prkachin, & Craig, 1977).

Concerning the discriminative capacity of the MPQ, Dubuisson and Melzack (1976), using a multiple discriminant analysis to identify diagnosis-specific clusters of pain descriptors, were able to generate reliably different clusters of pain descriptors for cancer pain, degenerative joint disease, menstrual pain, phantom-limb pain, arthritic pain, tooth pain, and post-herpic neuralgia. Using the MPQ, a discriminant analysis was correct in 77% in making a prediction of a patients clinical pain problem on the basis of verbal descriptors alone. Furthermore, the MPQ has been shown to be capable of discriminating between trigeminal neuralgia and atypical facial pain (Melzack et al., 1986).

Leavitt and Garron (1979) were able to discriminate low back pain patients with a positive somatic diagnosis from patients with the same complaint but a negative workup. Several other studies have confirmed the discriminative capacity of the MPQ (Chen & Treede, 1985; Gruska & Sessle, 1984; Hunter, 1983), while some have found that high pain intensity may obscure the MPQ's discriminative ability (Kremer & Atkinson, 1983; Reading, 1984).

Recently, Melzack, Katz, and Jeans (1985) demonstrated in an impressive way that it is a prejudice to impute pain patients on worker's compensation to report more severe levels of pain than noncompensation patients.

Some of the above-mentioned studies, however, have shown that modifications of the questionnaire may be necessary to suit the needs of the particular syndromes being studied.

The present questionnaire may be of use in the following circumstances: Communication may be facilitated in English-speaking countries for patients whose native language is German. Comparisons between data obtained from English and German-speaking patients may become feasible. Furthermore, multicentric cross-cultural studies involving verbal pain assessment may be conducted. We hope to have contributed to the development of such investigations.

References

Bradley, L.A., Prokop, C.K., Gentry, W.D., Van der Heide, L.H., & Prieto, E.J. (1981). Assessment of chronic pain. In C.K. Prokop & L.A. Bradley (Eds.), *Medical psychology: Contributions to behavioral medicine* (pp. 91–117). New York: Academic Press.

Byrne, M., Troy, A., Bradley, L. A., Marchisello, P.J., Geisinger, K.F., Van der Heide, L.H., & Prieto, E.J. (1982). Cross-validation of the factor structure of the McGill Pain Questionnaire. *Pain, 13,* 193–201.

Chen, A.C.N., & Hui, Y.L. (1984). *Headache in Taiwan: Assessment and characterization by a Chinese version of the McGill Pain Questionnaire and Bakel headache topographical chart.* Paper presented at the 4th World Pain Congress, Seattle, WA, Aug. 31–Sept. 5.

Chen, A.C.N., & Treede, R.-D. (1985). The McGill Pain Questionnaire in the assessment of phasic and tonic experimental pain: Behavioral evaluation of the "pain inhibiting pain" effect. *Pain, 22,* 67–79.

Crockett, D.J., Prkachin, K.M., & Craig, K.D. (1977). Factors of the language of pain in patient and volunteer groups. *Pain, 4,* 175–182.

Dubuisson, D., & Melzack, R. (1976). Classification of clinical pain descriptors by multiple group discriminant analysis. *Exp. Neurol., 51,* 480–487.

Gracely, R.H., McGrath, P., & Dubner, R. (1978). Validity and sensitivity of ratio scales of sensory and affective verbal pain descriptors: Manipulation of affect by diazepam. *Pain, 5,* 19–29.

Gruska, M., & Sessle, B.J. (1984). Applicability of the McGill Pain Questionnaire to the differentiation of "toothache" pain. *Pain, 19,* 49–57.

Harrison, A. (1988). Arabic pain words. *Pain, 32,* 239–250.

Hunter, M. (1983). The headache scale: A new approach to the assessment of headache pain based on pain descriptors. *Pain*, *16*, 361–373.

Huskisson, E.G. (1985). Visual analogue scales. In R. Melzack (Ed.), *Pain measurement and assessment* (pp. 33–37). New York: Raven Press.

Ketovuori, H., & Pöntinen, P.J. (1981). A pain vocabulary in Finnish – the Finnish pain questionnaire. *Pain*, *11*, 247–253.

Kiss, J., Müller, H., & Abel, M. (1987). The McGill Pain Questionnaire – German version. A study on cancer pain. *Pain*, *29*, 195–207.

Kremer, E.F., & Atkinson, J.H. (1981). Pain measurement: Construct validity of the affective dimension of the McGill Pain Questionnaire with chronic benign pain patients. *Pain*, *11*, 93–100.

Kremer, E.F., & Atkinson, J.H. (1983). Pain language as a measure of 8 affects in chronic pain patients. In R. Melzack (Ed.), *Pain measurement and assessment* (pp. 119–127). New York: Raven Press.

Lahuerta, J., Smith, B.A., & Martinez-Lage, J.M. (1982). An adaptation of the McGill Pain Questionnaire to the Spanish language. *Schmerz*, *3*, 132–134.

Leavitt, F., & Garron, D.C. (1979). Psychological disturbances and pain report differences in both organic and non-organic low back pain patients. *Pain*, *7*, 187–195.

Maiani, G., & Sanavio, E. (1985). Semantics of pain in Italy: the Italian version of the McGill Pain Questionnaire. *Pain*, *22*, 399–405.

McCreary, C., Turner, J., & Dawson, E. (1981). Principal dimension of the pain experience and psychological disturbance in chronic low back pain patients. *Pain*, *11*, 85–92.

Melzack, R., & Torgerson, W.S. (1971). On the language of pain. *Anesthesiology*, *34*, 50–60.

Melzack, R. (1975). The McGill Pain Questionnaire: major properties and scoring methods. *Pain*, *1*, 277–299.

Melzack, R. (1983). The measurement of pain experience. In S. Lipton & J. Miles (Eds.), *Persistent pain, Vol. 4* (pp. 173–193). London: Grune and Stratton.

Melzack, R., Katz, J., & Jeans, M.E. (1985). The role of compensation in chronic pain analysis using a new method of scoring the McGill Pain Questionnaire. *Pain*, *23*, 101–112.

Melzack, R., Terrence, C., Fromm, G., & Amsel, R. (1986). Trigeminal Neuralgia and atypical facial pain: Use of the McGill pain questionnaire for discrimination and diagnosis. *Pain*, *27*, 297–302.

Prieto, E.J., Hopson, L., Bradley, L.A., Byrne, M., Geisinger, K.F., Midax, D., & Marchisello, P.J. (1980). The language of low back pain: Factor structure of the McGill Pain Questionnaire. *Pain*, *8*, 11–19.

Prieto, E.J., & Geisinger, K.F. (1983). Factor-analytic studies of the McGill Pain Questionnaire, In R. Melzack (Ed.), *Pain measurement and assessment* (pp. 63–69). New York: Raven Press.

Radvila, A., Adler, R.H., Galeazzi, R.L., & Vorkauf, H. (1987). The development of a German language (Berne) pain questionnaire and its application in a situation causing acute pain. *Pain*, *28*, 185–195.

Reading, A.E. (1979). The internal structure of the McGill Pain Questionnaire in dysmenorrhoea patients. *Pain*, *7*, 353–358.

Reading, A.E. (1984). Testing pain mechanisms in persons pain. In P.D. Wall & R. Melzack (Eds.), *Textbook of pain* (pp. 195–204). Edinburgh: Churchill Livingstone.

Stein, C., Mendl, G., Pöppel, E., & Peter K. (1987). Semantics of pain in German: The development of a German version of the McGill Pain Questionnaire. *Pain Suppl. 4*, S. 161.

Stein, C., & Mendl, G. (1988). The German counterpart to the McGill Questionnaire. *Pain*, *32*, 251–255.

Turk, D.C., Rudy, T.E., & Salovey, P. (1985). The McGill Pain Questionnaire reconsidered: Confirming the factor structures and examining appropriate uses. *Pain*, *21*, 385–397.

SECTION C:
PSYCHOSOCIAL FACTORS IN PAIN PERCEPTION AND PAIN MANAGEMENT

Psychological Predictors of Therapy Outcome in Chronic Low Back Pain Patients

Monika Hasenbring

Following a critical discussion of test-psychological and experimental studies on the impact of psychological factors on acute or chronic pain, I present preliminary data from three of my own prospective studies. I examined a subgroup of low back pain patients, specifically patients with lumbar disc disease. I tried to predict therapy outcome by psychological and somatic factors. Results indicated that the *Beck Depression Inventory* (BDI) is the most significant predictor of persistent pain after discharge from the hospital. Results of the third study suggested that emotional and cognitive-behavioral reactions to chronic pain in everyday life are relevant predictors of persistent pain, and that somatic variables (e.g., pareses) are relevant predictors of the length of hospital stay. Results are discussed with reference to cognitive-behavioral concepts and learning theory.

According to the health services' 1983 annual statistics, gathered by the German Federal Ministry for Youth, Family and Health (Daten des Bundesgesundheitswesens, 1983), chronic low back pain is the most common reason for early retirement in employed men and the second most common reason in employed women. In the United States, the diagnosis "displacement of intervertebral disc" constitutes the second most common reason for disability in persons under the age of 50 (Kelsey, 1975). Irrespective of all organic causes, such as lumbar disc prolapse, inflammatory processes, and degenerative changes, the problems of persistent pain and immobilization are most important.

Here, hypotheses are formulated on the basis of a biopsychosocial model concerning the factors leading to chronicity of the bodily complaints. In prospective studies, these factors are then tested in view of the extent to which they can contribute to the prediction of a successful medical and/or psychological therapy. The results of empirical studies give point to the conclusion that psychological factors play an important role in the chronicity of low back pain disorders.

Three main points are discussed in this paper:

- psychological factors already examined in prospective studies as to their predictability of success in the treatment of low back pain patients;
- psychological factors examined in correlative or experimental studies in acute or chronic low back pain;
- psychological factors examined in our own prospective studies of lumbar disc patients.

Previous Prospective Studies

Since about the mid-1970s, a series of prospective studies using the *MMPI* have been carried out in which the attempt was made to predict the treatment outcome of low back pain patients (with or without organic causes; cf. Wiltse & Rocchio, 1975; McCreary, Turner, & Dawson, 1979; Oostdam & Duivenvoorden, 1983). In the most of these cases, patients with moderate or poor treatment results had higher scores for hysteria (Hy) and hypochondria (Hs) than did patients with more successful treatment. These results point to special attitudes in dealing with pain: It may be assumed that the fearful self-observation of bodily complaints is a factor leading to therapy resistance and to chronicity of complaints.

The role of an increased amount of depression as another predictor variable is explained even to a lesser extent. One can find a few prospective studies that are confirmed (McCreary, Turner, & Dawson, 1979; Kuperman, Osmon, Golden, & Blume, 1979), and those that are contradicted (Oostdam, & Duivenvoorden, 1983; Waring, Weisz, & Bailey, 1976). A frequent finding in the *MMPI* is the so-called "conversion-V," with a strong increase in the above-mentioned scale values of "Hy" and "Hs," and a smaller increase in depression (D). Also, to date it is still unclear (1) whether the partially increased D-values could be understood as an expression of a reaction toward pain that has already existed for years, (2) whether the "conversion-V" is the expression of a masked depression, or (3) whether the small increase in D-values is of no account (cf. Hasenbring & Ahrens, 1987). In this discussion, however, it should be observed that the *MMPI*-scale "D" assesses mainly the *affective* part of a state of depression, and not cognitive or somatic parts. This will be reconsidered further below.

Two critical points should be mentioned with regard to the results from the *MMPI*:

- groups with good and poor treatment outcomes show significant differences in the scales Hy, Hs, and D. On the other hand, there is such a large overlap between groups that an individual predictability still remains uncertain.
- the *MMPI* is very long, and most of the items are not reasonable for patients suffering from pain. Therefore, it is only partially suitable as a screening instrument.

Melzack and Wall's (1965) Gate-Control Theory stresses, in a complex psychophysiological model, the role of emotional and cognitive components of pain experience. In a series of general (*McGill Pain Questionnaire*, Melzack, 1975; Melzack & Torgerson, 1971) and illness-specific scales (e.g., *Back Pain Classification Scale*, Leavitt, 1983) different aspects of pain quality can be assessed: sensory ("pulsing," "burning"), affective ("dangerous"), and cognitive-evaluative ("annoying," "unbearable") aspects. Some of these studies had shown the usefulness of these scales in distinguishing "functional" and "organic" back pain.

Even today the attempt to predict therapy outcome has not succeeded (Dzioba & Doxey, 1984).

Correlative or Experimental Studies

In the meantime, there are quite many empirical studies investigating the influence of psychological variables upon subjectively experienced intensity of pain and pain behavior. Most of these are based on psychological or psychophysiological theories tested during acute pain. It might be tested whether these factors also could predict the treatment outcome of chronic low back pain.

Cognitive Factors in Pain Experience

In particular Roskies and Lazarus (1980) as well as Meichenbaum and Turk (1976) have emphasized the important role that cognitions play in the pain experience. In numerous experimental studies concerning acute pain, the impact of negative cognitions (e.g., "catastrophizing"), positive cognitions ("positive self-statements"), and distractive cognitions ("imagery," "attention diversion") on pain experience has been proven (Turk, Meichenbaum, & Genest, 1983). Rosenstiel and Keefe (1983) developed a questionnaire to assess cognitive strategies for coping with pain in chronic low back pain patients. They found that cognitive strategies of "diversion" and "reinterpretation" are associated with a high degree of functional impairment, whereas cognitions of "catastrophizing" are associated with a higher amount of fear and depression. Here, interesting differences are shown in the adaptability of cognitive strategies for acute and chronic pain. These differences should be clarified within prospective studies.

Emotional Factors of Pain Experience

Gentry and Bernal (1974), among others, stress the role of emotional reactions during pain within the classical conditioning model. If the perception of a painful stimulus is accompanied by fear, and if a connection exists between pain and movement, then this leads to an avoidance of movements and to a decrease of pain. Here a dangerous cycle sets in, which leads to an increased immobilization in everyday life. To our knowledge, there is no questionnaire available that assesses specific emotional reactions during pain, and that could be used in patients suffering from chronic pain. The above-mentioned cycle is not yet empirically proven.

Overt Pain Behavior Patterns

Fordyce (1976), as well as Keefe and coworkers (Keefe, 1982; Keefe & Gil, 1986) have directed attention toward the numerous behavioral patterns individuals use to communicate their pain to their spouse or other persons. These behaviors, termed "pain behaviors," include verbal descriptions of pain, pain medication intake as well as specific body postures and facial expressions indicative of pain. Low back pain patients, for example, communicate their pain by changing their posture, by using a cane, by groaning, by twisting their faces, etc. The operant conditioning model describes how patients may learn that such pain behaviors are followed by different reinforcing processes. Drastic consequences leading to early retirement from unpleasant working conditions are the ultimate results of a chronicity process; more frequent and milder consequences are, for example, special attention and care from spouses, instrumental help in everyday life, or the avoidance of unpleasant social contact. White and Sanders (1986), in a striking experimental study, showed the influence of positive support toward pain behavior on subjectively experienced pain intensity. However, up to now there are no prospective studies proving the significance of overt pain behavior and operant processes for the chronicity of pain.

Psychodynamic Model

Within psychodynamic concepts, characteristics of personality and specific conflicts of LBP patients were described for pain without any definite organic diagnosis. Accordingly, Fleck (1975) described 50 patients with radicular syndrome as having a compulsory helping attitude, excessive work enthusiasm, and not being able to enjoy pleasure. Critical situations in which back pain frequently appears are characterized by a conflict between the challenge of withstanding and unconscious wishes of revolt or of giving up. These conflicts are supposed to induce muscular hypertension. Kütemeyer and Schultz (1985) also described these attitudes in patients with lumbar-sciatic pain from an inpatient setting.

Psychophysiological Concepts

In a stress-strain hypothesis, it is supposed that heavy stress leads to autonomic arousal and increased muscle activity; repeated or continued muscle strain leads to pain through ischaemia and release of biochemical substances. Flor, Turk, and Birbaumer (1985) showed that low back pain patients reacted to personally relevant stress stimuli by a specific activity of the paraspinal muscles. As far as we know, no prospective study exists in LBP patients in which the degree of individual stress or psychophysiological response patterns have been used as predictors for treatment outcome (see also Teufel & Traue, in this volume).

Our Own Prospective Studies

In three consecutive prospective studies, we examined a subgroup of LBP patients, namely, patients with lumbar disc prolapse. We tried to predict treatment outcome (both conservative therapy and surgery) by psychological and somatic variables. In the following, I give an overview of these three studies. I would particularely like to point out that we are now only at the beginning of the data analysis for Studies 2 and 3, so that this allows only a first possible indication. To keep with the theme of this paper, I will put the main emphasis on psychological predictors.

The goal of the first study (Hasenbring & Ahrens, 1987) was to test the predictive value of the variables depression (via trait and state variables) and experience of pain. In accordance to the clinical-neurological data at discharge, we compared patients still complaining of pain but without a serious organic diagnosis (Group A) with the remaining ones (Group B). We assumed that Group A already had higher pretreatment values on the scales FPI-3 (depression), BDI, and on the Hoppe scales "pain-suffering" and "pain-fear" (Table 1).

Table 1. Results of the first study (Hasenbring & Ahrens, 1987).

	Group	n	M	S
FPI−3 (depression)	A	10	2.40	0.97
	B	28	1.93	0.87
BDI** (depression)	A	10	11.60	6.02
	B	28	5.32	4.05
HOPPE- anxiety	A	10	2.08	1.32
	B	28	2.22	1.71
suffering*	A	10	3.35	1.34
	B	28	4.62	1.23
sharpness	A	10	3.08	1.56
	B	28	3.08	1.26
rhythmic	A	10	1.69	1.23
	B	28	2.03	1.23

* $p\ 0.05$
** $p\ 0.01$
FPI-3: Freiburger Persönlichkeitsinventar Skala Depressivität.
BDI: Beck Depression Inventory
HOPPE: Quality of pain
M: mean
S: standard deviation

The only significant predictor in this study was the BDI, with a predictibility of 86%. Patients with persistent pain after discharge had higher scores on the BDI (before treatment) than patients without pain or with only minimal pain. There was no difference between Group A and Group B in the demographic variables age and sex, and in the somatic variables duration of pain and number of previous operations. We tested the group differences by t-test for independent samples under consideration of alpha adjustments. The difference in the Hoppe scale "pain-suffering" was contrary to our expectation.

Moreover, we differentiated the total-score of the BDI into four factors (Kammer, 1983), two cogitive factors called "self-punishing" and "feelings of guilt," one somatic factor called "somatic complaints," and one affective factor called "sadness" (see Table 2). The results show that significant group differences are primarily based on the factor "somatic complaints" and on the factor "self-punishing." There are no differences in the affective part of the depression scale "sadness" and in the other cognitive part "feelings of guilt."

Table 2. Results of the first study. Mean differences between group A and group B, BDI Scales.

BDI-Scales	group	n	M	S
self punishing*	A	10	2.00	1.56
	B	28	0.75	1.01
somatic complaints**	A	10	4.70	2.11
	B	28	2.11	2.04
sadness	A	10	1.10	2.18
	B	28	0.54	1.14
feelings of guilt	A	10	1.80	1.48
	B	28	1.14	1.35

* p 0.05   ** p 0.01   M: mean   S: standard deviation

In the second study (Hasenbring, Ahrens, & Marienfeld, in preparation), we intended to replicate the results for the BDI and to compare them with other state (DS, v. Zerssen, 1977) and trait variables (*Gießen-Test*, Beckmann & Richter, 1981). In addition, for the first time we included Hoppe's scale (Hoppe, 1985) for assessing overt pain behavior. This scale consists of 27 self-statement items which describe different overt pain behaviors. The criteria assessing treatment outcome was set up as in the former study. The only significant group difference was found in the BDI and the Hoppe scale "motoric/facial pain expression" (Table 3). Patients in group A were more depressive and showed more expressive pain behavior than those in group B. For this study as well as for Study 3, we are still carrying out multiple regression analyses, in order to examine the relative predictability of the individual variables and supressor effects.

Table 3. Results of the second prospective study (Hasenbring, Ahrens, & Marienfeld, in preparation). N = 41 (21).

	Group	n	M	S
Depression				
BDI**	A	5	10.2	5.3
	B	15	4.1	3.4
DS-Zerssen	A	5	6.2	2.7
	B	16	4.8	1.7
GT	A	5	25.2	5.9
	B	16	22.6	7.1
Pain Perception				
HOPPE: anxiety	A	7	1.7	0.7
	B	19	1.6	1.2
suffering	A	7	2.8	1.4
	B	19	3.4	1.9
sharpness	A	7	2.4	1.6
	B	19	2.2	0.4
rhythmic	A	7	1.5	1.2
	B	19	1.6	0.7
Pain Behavior				
HOPPE: avoiding	A	7	1.7	0.6
	B	19	1.4	0.3
control	A	7	1.8	0.5
	B	19	1.7	0.4
distraction	A	7	1.6	0.4
	B	19	1.4	0.3
motoric*	A	7	3.0	0.7
	B	19	2.1	0.6

* p 0.05
** p 0.01
BDI: Beck Depression Inventory
DS: Depressions-Skala von Zerssen
GT: Gießen-Test
M: mean
S: standard deviation

In the third study, we used several self-developed, as yet unpublished questionnaires concerning cognitive, emotional, and behavioral aspects of pain experience. Based on Lazarus and Launier's (1978) theory of stress, these instruments assess emotional reactions during everyday life situations of pain experience (ERSS), cognitive reactions (KRSS), and coping reactions (CRSS) (Hasenbring, in preparation). An example is shown on Table 4.

Table 4. Items from ERSS Scale (emotional reactions in pain situations).

When I'm in pain I feel . . . .

	each time						never
. . . depressed	6	5	4	3	2	1	0
. . . irritated	6	5	4	3	2	1	0
. . . nevertheless happy	6	5	4	3	2	1	0
. . . angry	6	5	4	3	2	1	0

Here, patients describe how they feel when they consciously experience pain. For each emotion they indicate on a 7-point scale, ranging from "never" to "each time," how often this has occurred within the last 14 days.

We employed data from 147 chronic pain patients in factor analysis and item analysis. For the scale ERSS, we extracted, on the basis of a Varimax rotation and Eigenvalues 1.00, a clear cut 3-factor solution with the factors "depression," "anger," and "raised mood" (Table 5). The three factors accounted for 62% of the variance. The internal consistency (Cronbach's Alpha) was 0.89, 0.79, and 0.79.

Table 5. ERSS Scale (emotional reactions in pain situations). Results of factor analysis (varimax-rotation).

factor	% of Var	Alpha	N of Items
F1 Depression	40.4	.89	8
F2 Anger	7.6	.79	3
F3 Happiness	14.2	.79	3
Total	62.2		

For the KRSS scale, we extracted 6 factors: "helplessness/hopelessness," "barrier," "catastrophizing," "minimizing," "psychic causal attribution," and "coping signal." The six factors accounted for 59% of the variance. Coefficients of reliability are satisfactory (Table 6).

For the CRSS scale, we extracted nine factors because we wanted to assess individual coping strategies in a differentiated mode (Table 7). Eight factors accounted for less then 10% of the common variance. Nevertheless, we decided to use these factors because they allow a meaningful interpretation. Values for internal consistency are satisfactory except for two scales (F7 and F10).

The following predictors resulted from the third study: Up to now we defined two criteria for treatment outcome: (1) the length of hospital stay, in days; (2) the intensity of pain 6 weeks after discharge (8-point scale).

Table 6. KRSS Scale (cognitive reactions in pain situations). Results of factor analysis (varimax rotation).

Factor	% of Var	Alpha	N of Items
F1 Help/hopelessness	31.8	.89	9
F2 Barrier	8.9	.89	7
F3 Catastrophizing	5.9	.79	4
F4 Minimizing	4.8	.66	5
F5 Psychological attribution	4.0	.87	2
F6 Coping signal	3.5	.69	3
Total	58.9		

Alpha: Cronbach's Alpha

Table 7. CRSS Scale (coping strategies in pain situations). Results of factor analysis (varimax rotation).

Factor	% of Var	Alpha	N of items
F1 Avoidance of social activity	14.9	.86	9
F2 Overt behavior	8.2	.78	6
F3 Job interruption	4.5	.77	3
F4 Search for social support	4.1	.74	5
F5 Active distraction	3.7	.81	3
F6 Avoidance of exertion	3.4	.75	4
F7 Ignoring	3.2	.66	4
F8 To stick it out	3.2	.74	6
F9 Passive distraction	2.9	.59	3
Total	48.1		

Alpha: Cronbach's Alpha

The sample of this study consists of 85 lumbar disc patients before surgery. With respect to the first criterion, the BDI and the neurological data (pareses) have been proven to be significant predictors. Patients with a BDI score greater than "10" and/or a pareses had a mean score of 21 days in the hospital, and patients with a BDI score below "10" and/or no pareses, a mean of 13 days. The coping scales ERSS, KRSS, and CRSS turned out to be significant predictors for the second criterion, pain intensity 6 weeks after discharge. Patients with persistent pain had higher scores on scales "depression" and "anger" (ERSS), "helplessness/ hopelessness" and "barrier" (KRSS), and on the scales "ignoring" and "to stick it out" from CRSS did than patients without pain or with minimal pain.

Discussion

Up to now there have been very few theoretically founded psychometric studies that contribute to the prediction of persistent pain in lumbar disc patients. In our studies we examined for the first time both emotional and cognitive-behavioral factors as predictors of persistent pain in lumbar disc patients. The impact of these factors on the experience of pain has been proven in numerous experimental studies concerning acute pain. All three studies confirmed the role of depression as a relevant predictor of treatment success. Moreover, several learning and cognitive factors are shown to be relevant psychological predictors for the problem of persistent pain and for length of hospital stay, too.

In the first and second study, the BDI turned out to be the most important predictor for persistent pain at discharge. In both studies the accuracy of predictability was more than 80%. These results are largely due to the somatic and cognitive aspects of a depressive state, and not to the affective ones. It still remains unclear whether the raised BDI scores are to be understood as a reaction to pain experience or as an aspect of "masked depression." Here, only a clinical psychological interview can give further information (Hasenbring, 1987).

Furthermore, in the second study, "overt pain behavior" proved to be a relevant predictor of treatment success. Patients with persistent pain clearly admitted that they change their posture more often, they groan, twist their faces or rub the painful areas more often than do patients with no more pain. This result is to be interpreted especially in the light of the operant conditioning model (Fordyce, 1976; Keefe & Gil, 1986).

Preliminary data analysis from the third study proved that the BDI and the somatic findings (pareses) are relevant predictors for the length of hospital stay (cf. Rosenstiel & Gross, 1986). In addition, the newly developed scales for coping with pain contributed to the prediction of persistent pain 6 weeks after discharge. Patients with persistent pain were characterized, on the one hand, by higher scores on the scales "depression" and "anger" (from ERSS) as well as "helplessness/hopelessness" and "barrier" (from KRSS), and on the other hand, by higher scores in the scales "to ignore" and "to stick it out" (from CRSS). This can be interpreted as a conflict between cognitive and emotional pain experience and coping strategies. On the one hand, patients with persistent pain try to ignore their pain and to stick it out; on the other hand, they experience their pain as a barrier. They are more angry in pain situations or they feel more helplessness/hopelessness than patients without persistent pain after treatment. In this conflict such patients lack positive coping strategies like relaxation techniques, which would lead to reduced muscle tension. It can be assumed that this conflict results in heightened muscle tension and more pain.

Moreover, results of the third study suggest that the organic findings (e.g., pareses) are important predictors for the length of hospital stay but not for the occurrence of persistent pain. Therefore, in further studies we have to assess both organic and psychological data as predictors, and to differentiate several criteria of treatment success, such as "length of hospital stay," "pain quality and intensity," "occurrence of somatic complaints after surgery," "medication intake," and "return to work".

References

Beckmann, D., & Richter, H.E. (1972). *Gießen-Test. Handbuch.* Bern: Hans Huber.
Dzioba, R.B., & Doxey, N.C. (1984). A prospective investigation into the orthopaedic and psychologic predictors of outcome of first lumbar surgery following industrial injury. *Spine, 9,* 614—623.
Fleck, H.E. (1975). Über psychodynamische Faktoren bei Wurzelreizerscheinungen. *Zeitschrift für Psychosomatische Medizin und Psychoanalyse, 21,* 118—128.
Flor, H., Turk, D., & Birbaumer, N. (1985). Assessment of stress-related psychophysiological reactions in chronic back pain patients. *Journal of Consulting and Clinical Psychology, 53,* 354—364.
Fordyce, W.E. (1976). Behavioral methods for chronic pain and illness. St. Louis: Mosby.
Gentry, W.D., & Bernal, G.A. (1977). Chronic pain. In R.B. Williams & W.D. Gentry (Eds.), *Behavioral approaches to medical treatment* (pp. 173—182). Cambridge, MA: Ballinger.
Hasenbring, M. (1987). *Das Kieler Interview zur subjektiven Situation KISS bei Schmerzpatienten.* Paper presented at the first workshop on "pain measurement," Mainz, FRG.
Hasenbring, M. (1988). *The development of three scales to assess cognitive, emotional and behavioral reactions to chronic pain.* Poster presentation at the International Conference of Health Psychology, Trier, FRG, May.
Hasenbring, M., & Ahrens, S. (1987). Depressivität, Schmerzwahrnehmung und Schmerzerleben bei Patienten mit lumbalem Bandscheibenvorfall, Psychotherapie. *Psychosomatik und Medizinische Psychologie, 37,* 149—155.
Hasenbring, M., Ahrens, S., & Marienfeld, G. (in preparation). *Zur Vorhersage des Behandlungserfolges bei Patienten mit bandscheibenbedingtem Lumbo-Ischias-Syndrom. Eine Replikationsstudie.*
Hoppe, F. (1985). Zur Faktorenstruktur von Schmerzerleben und Schmerzverhalten bei chronischen Schmerzpatienten. *Diagnostika, 31,* 70—78.
Kammer, D. (1983). Eine Untersuchung der psychometrischen Eigenschaften des deutschen Beck-Depressionsinventars (BDI). *Diagnostika, 24,* 48—60.
Keefe, F.J. (1982). Behavioral assessment and treatment of chronic pain: Current status and futur directions. *Journal of Consulting and Clinical Psychology, 50,* 896911.
Keefe, F.J., & Gil, K.M. (1986). Behavioral concepts in the analysis of chronic pain syndromes. *Journal of Consulting and Clinical Psychology, 54,* 776—783.
Kelsey, J.L. (1975). An epidemiological study of acute herniated lumbar intervertebral discs. *Rheumatology and Rehabilitation, 14,* 144—159.

Kuperman, S., Osmon, D., Golden, C., & Blume, H. (1979). Prediction of neurosurgical results by psychological evaluation. *Perceptual and Motor Skills, 48,* 311—315.

Kütemeyer, M., & Schultz, U. (1986). Psychosomatik des Lumbago-Ischias-Syndroms. In v. Uexküll, T. (Ed.), *Psychosomatische Medizin* (p. 838). Munich/Baltimore: Urban & Schwarzenberg.

Lazarus, R.S., & Launier, R. (1978). Stress-related transactions between person and environment. In L.A. Pervin & M. Lewis (Eds.), *Perspectives in interactional psychology* (pp. 287—327). New York: Plenum Press.

Leavitt, F. (1983). Detecting psychological disturbance using verbal pain measurement: The back pain classification scale. In R. Melzack (Ed.), *Pain measurement and assessment* (pp. 79—84). New York: Raven Press.

McCreary, C., Turner, J., & Dawson, E. (1981). Principal dimensions of the pain experience and psychological disturbance in chronic low back pain patients. *Pain, 11,* 85—92.

Meichenbaum, D.H., & Turk, D.C. (1976). The cognitive-behavioral management of anxiety, anger, and pain. In P.O. Davidson (Ed.), *The behavioral management of anxiety, depression and pain.* New York: Brunner/Mazel.

Melzack, R., & Wall, P.D. (1965). Pain mechanisms: A new theory. *Science, 50,* 971—979.

Melzack, R., & Torgerson, W.S. (1971). On the language of pain. *Anaesthesiology, 34,* 50—59.

Melzack, R. (1975). The McGill Pain Questionnaire: Major properties and scoring methods. *Pain, 1,* 277—299.

Oostdam, E.M.M., & Duivenvoorden, H.J. (1983). Predictability of the result of surgical intervention in patients with low back pain. *Journal of Psychosomatic Research, 27,* 273—281.

Rosenstiel, A.K., & Keefe, F.J. (1983). The use of coping strategies in chronic low back pain patients: Relationships to patient characteristics and current adjustment. *Pain, 17,* 33—44.

Rosenstiel, A.K., & Gross, A. (1986). The effect of coping strategies on the relief of pain following surgical intervention for lower back pain. *Psychosomatic Medicine, 48,* 229—241.

Roskies, E., & Lazarus, R.S. (1980). Coping theory and the teaching of coping skills. In P.O. Davidson & S.M. Davidson (Eds.), *Behavioral medicine: Changing health life styles.* New York: Brunner/Mazel.

Turk, D.C., Meichenbaum, D., & Genest, M. (1983). *Pain and behavioral medicine.* New York: Guilford Press.

Waring, E.M., Weisz, G.M., & Bailey, S.E. (1976). Predictive factors of the treatment of low back pain by surgical intervention. *Advances in Pain Research and Therapy, 1,* 939—942.

White, B., & Sanders, S.H. (1986). The influence on patients' pain intensity ratings of antecedent reinforcement of pain talk or well talk. *Journal of Behavior Therapy & Experimental Psychiatry, 17,* 155—159.

Wiltse, L.L., & Rocchio, P.D. (1975). Preoperative psychological tests as predictors of success of chemonucleolysis in the treatment of the low back syndrome. *Journal of Bone and Joint Surgery, 57,* 478—483.

Zerssen, D.v. (1977). *Die Depressivitätsskala.* Weinheim: Beltz.

Psychological Profiles of Chronic Pain Patients and Factors Predisposing to the Development of Pain-Induced Psychological Disorders

Peter Marschall, Ingrid Bowdler, Friedbert Rieth

This paper examines personality traits and impairment of social activity in chronic pain patients. It is assumed that abnormal behavior is the result of a pain history rather than a predisposition. The psychological profiles of pain patients such as personality traits, symptom reporting, and depression, are compared with normative data.

Chronic pain with either headache or backache was studied. Multiple regression analysis revealed that chronification of pain leads to an increase of symptom reporting, particularily in the musculo-skeletal system.

Pain patients are characterized by having many somatic complaints and a marked depression. Other psychological traits failed to describe a pain profile. Backache patients had the least of all bodily symptoms. They have been found well apart from headache patients. Subjective data based on routine psychological testing could not identify any type of psychological disorder. Differential aspects are described.

This study focuses on patients with either chronic headache or backache. The psychological characteristics of these patients have often been assessed and compared with the normal population, but, by and large, statistical analysis has failed to show significant differences. In 1937, Wolff presented a now classical description of typical migraine patients as being ambitious, having high ideals with respect to their own person, and as being drawn by social prestige. Even today, some specialists agree with this assessment. Haas (1985) pointed out that the perfectionism, exactness, and responsibility of these patients are assets that are especially valued in the work setting. Geissler (1980) suggested, however, that it is precisely these personality traits which give rise to specific conflicts when these patients fail to achieve the high ideals they have set for themselves. These authors regard such characteristics as typical for the migraine patient. Peters (1983) even goes so far as to identify a "Typus migrainicus," but this is a point of view that cannot be accepted without criticism. The above-mentioned descriptions are based on only small numbers of patients without control group observations, and are therefore of questionable value. Study of the literature nevertheless shows that the uncertainty raised by the suggestion that migraine patients differ from completly healthy persons in a constant manner has not been laid to rest. The question also remains as to whether any of the psychological changes found in chronic pain patients are a result of the long-acting and/or recurring pain experience itself (Larbig, 1982; Knapp, 1983).

Patients with muscle tension headache are also presumed to have abnormal behavior patterns and an abnormal view of themselves and their surroundings.

Friedman (1979) found that tension headache is more commonly associated with anxiety than would be expected by chance. A deficiency in the ability to express emotions in situations giving rise to anger and aggression has been correlated with this type of headache, as has the presence of depression (Beyme, 1976; Holroyd & Andrasik, 1978; Weatherhead, 1980; Traue et al., 1985). In a review of the literature, Kröner (1982) summarized the psychological characteristics of tension headache patients as follows: general emotional instability, anxiety, inability to withstand emotional pressure, reduced ability to express aggression, tendency to conform with what is perceived as being "normal," and a punctilious tidiness. Bell et al. (1983) added to this list an above-average degree of irritability, a desire to be dependent on others, and an increased tendency to develop psychosomatic disorders of all kinds. These characteristics are derived from both "clinical" impressions and psychological testing. Most studies have being carried out using the MMPI and the Eysenck Personality Questionnaire (EPQ).

A number of studies (Kudrow & Sutkus, 1979; Andrasik et al., 1982; Sternbach, 1983) have used the MMPI to assess abnormal behavior in chronic pain patients. These authors have also compared patients with different headache types using this method. Although not absolutely consistent, a so-called "conversion V," i.e., high test values in the first scale (hypochondria) and third scale (hysteria) associated with a mild degree of depression (second scale), or a so-called "neurotic triad" (above differences together with a markedly increased depression score) was frequently found to be present. In his study on random samples of a hospital population, Andrasik et al. (1982) in particular was able to find evidence of this neurotic triad. These authors also compared the results obtained with their headache patients with those of a symptom-free control group and found that in addition to the above findings, the MMPI scales 6 (paranoia) and 7 (pychasthenia) were significantly different between the groups. No significant difference was found between the patients of the various headache groups, but they could be ranked in order of their degree of variation from the norm. Here, it was found that, compared to the other groups, the personality traits of migraine patients differed least from healthy controls, but showed a tendency to have a larger number of somatic symptoms. In addition to this tendency, patients with a combined headache were characterized by mild depression, a tendency toward worrying, and pessimism. Those patients diagnosed as having muscle tension headache had the most remarkedly abnormal results on a number of psychological scales. They, however, were the patients with the most stressful life styles.

The descriptions of a typical headache patient are therefore quite varied, as has been pointed out by Blanchard, Andrasik, and Arena (1984) in a survey of 19 studies.

In a study using the Eysenck Personality Questionnaire (EPQ) carried out on headache sufferers who where not undergoing any form of treatment, Philips (1976) found no differences between the various headache types or between the headache group and a normal population. These results indicate that psychological changes are the *result* rather than the course of the painful disorder (Blaszcynski, 1984; Franz et al., 1986; Köhler, Kraus, & Vanselow, 1987).

Franz et al. (1986) compared the *MMPI* profile of patients with chronic headache to those with chronic low back pain. Hypochrondria, depression, and hysteria were significantly higher in both pain groups than in the controls, whereby the two pain groups had very similar values. One of the reasons for regarding chronic low back pain as a psychophysiological and psychosocial problem is that such patients do not have a higher incidence of degenerative changes on X-ray than do a symptom-free normal population (Flor & Turk, 1984). Just as is the case for headache patients, clinical observation, psychological testing, and experimental investigations have been carried out on this group of patients. Turk and Flor (1984) described the typical low back pain patient as having the desire to run away from unpleasent situations. Not being able to translate this wish into action is suggested to result in an increase in muscle tone and hence in pain. These investigators report an increase in the height of action potential of the paravertebal muscles in a group of 65 patients with low back pain and cervical paravertebral symptoms when placed in unpleasant situations. When conversation is turned to topics leading to feelings of uncertainty and aggression, EMG recordings increase, in particular in the musculature of the lower back. In the 1950s the poor results of surgical interventions in this group of patients led American orthopaedic surgeons to try and identify which patients probably had functional disorders and should not be subjected to operation.

Hanvik (1951) developed a shortened form of the *MMPI* with 25 items, called the "Low Back Pain Scale." In a thorough review of the literature, Murray (1982) concludes that it is extremely difficult to differentiate between "organic" and "functional" back pain on the basis of *MMPI* profiles. The profiles obtained were not sufficiently characteristic to be able to recognize a set pattern, and are thus not recommended (Rosen, Frymoyer, & Clements, 1980; Love & Peck, 1987; Turk & Rudy, 1987). The back pain classification scale, which is based on the *McGill Pain Questionnaire* (Leavitt & Sweet, 1983), has also been used to try to differentiate between these subgroups. In other studies using the *MMPI* in which prediction of treatment outcome was attempted, Love and Peck (1987) were not able to define a "low back pain" or a "chronic pain" personality profile.

Just as in the headache group, it remains at present unresolved if and to what degree chronic pain per se results in psychological changes in low back pain patients. McGill et al. (1983) report that increasing duration of illness as well as the number of hospital stays and operations contribute to pain-induced psychological disorders.

One of the aims of this study was to test this assumption by comparing the duration of pain as the criterion with the "conversion V" as dependent variable, i.e., with the presence of a large number of somatic symptoms (hypochondria), and an increased sensitivity toward "disturbances" and a variety of ever-changing functional symptoms (hysteria as defined in the *MMPI*). In addition, we assessed the "neurotic triad" as characterized by a marked depression in contrast to a mild depression in the "conversion V." Our samples were taken from patients presenting to a pain clinic, and in formulating our hypotheses we have therefore concentrated on the findings obtained during routine examination of these patients.

Pain-induced disorders cannot be adequately assessed by defining personality traits only. Pain is a burden that can markedly impair social activity, whether in respect to family life, sexual activity, leisure time, or professional activities. In order to assess whether these factors are causal in the development of pain-induced disorders, we used a battery of tests that assesses not only the patients' personality traits, but also their social status and social activities.

First Hypothesis

The duration of a chronic pain patient's history determines the extent to which psychological changes develop. The longer the duration of the pain complaint, the more marked are the associated psychosomatic changes (hypochondria, hysteria, depression). Chronic pain also leads to restrictions within the whole sphere of social activities, which are consequently felt to be a burden rather than a pleasure.

The attempt has been made in a large number of studies to differentiate between various types of diagnoses on the basis of psychological testing, usually without success (Franz et al., 1986). A tendency toward higher neuroticism scores is reported, migraine patients having a profile fairly similar to healthy controls, tension headache patients having higher scores, while headache patients with the a diagnoses of a conversion neurosis had the highest neuroticism scores.

We presume that the type of pain diagnosis made is not relevant to the personality traits subsequently found.

Second Hypothesis

Thus, personality traits and indicators of stress such as changes in social activity and status cannot be used to differentiate between the following four diagnoses: vascular headache, muscle tension headache, combined headache, low back pain.

A number of articles suggest that women report more somatic complaints than men (Brähler & Scheer, 1983; Pennebaker, 1982). We would therefore expect this difference to be mirrored in a chronic pain population. Women suffer some 2 to 4 times more frequently from migraine (Knapp, 1983). This difference is smaller amongst those suffering from tension headache and backache.

Third Hypothesis

Thus, analogous to the reports in the psychosomatic literature which describe women as having a larger number of somatic complaints than men, female chronic pain patients have a greater number of somatic symptoms than their male counterparts. They are more abnormal in the psychosomatic sense. No hypothesis can be put forward concerning any other personality traits.

That family life is correlated to the presence of illness is described in a review article by Sterling and Eyer (1981), who found that the risk of illness and of developing a chronic disability is greatest for persons living alone. This risk is slightly higher for unmarried, higher for divorced, and higher still for widowed persons. The authors largely drew their data from epidemiological studies on cardiovascular disease and cancer.

Fourth Hypothesis

The developement of a chronic pain state is dependent on the degree of social support experienced by the individual. In contrast to social activities occurring within a private sphere, such as sexual activity, status within the family determines whether chronic pain develops. As one of the characteristics of pain in this disorder we would expect to find a reduction in social activities as assessed by the "social support scale."

Our data are derived from standard psychodiagnostic testing and a written social history. All our patients suffered from chronic pain. The results obtained were scored from the following questionnaires: a personality trait test, a list of gemeralized complaints, and a paranoia-depression scale.

Methods

Subjects

All the patients part taking in this study were suffering from chronic pain syndromes and had presented to the pain clinic of Ulm University. In order to be included in this study, the pain had to be of nonmalignant origin and present for least three months. The 309 cases included in the study were placed into one of the following 6 diagnostic groups:

— vascular headache: 65 patients (21.0%)
— tension headache: 53 patients (17.2%)
— combined headache: 20 patients (6.5%)
— conversion neurosis headache: 3 patients (1.0%)
— low back pain: 32 patients (10.4%)
— other pain syndromes: 136 patients (44.0%)

The diagnosis of a headache subsequent to conversion neurosis was only made in three cases, so that this group was too small to be included in the study. In order to be able to assess the effect of marital and familial status on the development of pain-induced disorders, all 306 chronic pain patients were included.

Further statistical calculations were carried out only on those patients who had headache or low back pain.

Procedure

A routine and a pain-oriented case history was taken from all patients, who were examined by a doctor experienced in pain clinic practice. All earlier case notes, including those of other clinics, were obtained. An interim diagnosis was made at the first presentation, and further diagnostic measures were initiated where appropriate. All of the patients were then seen by a medical psychologist, who carried out a standard interview in which, amongst other things, profession, family status, personal contacts, self-efficacy, appriceation of bodily functions, and emotions and the hopes placed on various types of therapy was explored. Then the psychological questionnaires were filled out. When both the medically and psychologically oriented results had been gathered, the case was discussed in an interdisciplinary pain conference, where the doctor treating the patient, the pain therapy consultant, the psychologist, and, when necessary, specialists from other disciplines discussed the case in order to reach a definite diagnosis and to formulate a plan of management.

The following tests were used for the psychological assessment:

– the *Biographisches Inventar zur Diagnose von Verhaltensstörungen* (Biographical Inventory for the Diagnosis of Behavior Abnormalities) (BIV) (Jäger et al., 1976). This test was designed to describe the personality traits of a subject and to supply additional information about the patient's biography and his or her present social situation. There are "yes" or "no" 97 items which describe 8 different characteristics: familiar interactions, self-efficacy, social status, parental upbringing, neuroticism, social activities, psychophysical constitution, and extraversion.

– The *Gießener Beschwerdebogen* (Gießen Symptom Assessment)(GBB) (Brähler & Scheer, 1983), consisting of 57 items. The degree to which the various symptoms are present is marked on a Likert-scale from "none" to "marked." Twenty-four of the items are included in one of four assessment scales: exhaustion, indigestion, musculo-skeletal complaints, and cardiac symptoms. The fifth assessment-scale, "the burden of the somatic symptoms," is the summation of the previous 24 items. After transformation of the raw data, the results can be compared with samples drawn from the normal healthy population and with patient diagnosed as being psychosomatically ill.

– The *Paranoid-Depressivitäts-Skala* (Paranoia Depression Scale) (PDS) (v. Zerssen & Köhler, 1976), which assesses if and to what degree a depression or paranoia are present. A subscale "illness denial" looks at the tendency to play down symptoms of illness or, on the contrary, to complain in somatic terms of psychological disturbances. Forty-two subquestions are answered on a Likert-scale, normal values being based on a healthy population already known.

Results

In our first hypothesis we postulated a correlation between the duration of pain (chronification) and neuroticism, which we operationalized with the "conversion-V" (hypochondria, hysteria, and a mild depression) and/or the "neurotic triad" (hypochondria, hysteria, and a marked depression). According to the hypochondriasis concept, we expected a higher score for complaint reporting in our *Gießen Complaints Questionnaire,* and in the scale "psychophysical constitution" of the BIV. We also expected a higher neuroticism score in this test. Depression was assessed by the *Paranoid-Depression Scale.* In this sense, the algogenic psychosyndrome can be positively correlated with the duration of pain.

We separated the duration of pain into 4 classes, from less than 6 months (6.2% of patients) up to 5 years (58.6% of patients). Figure 1 indicates percentage and numbers of pain patients in relation to the duration of their complaints.

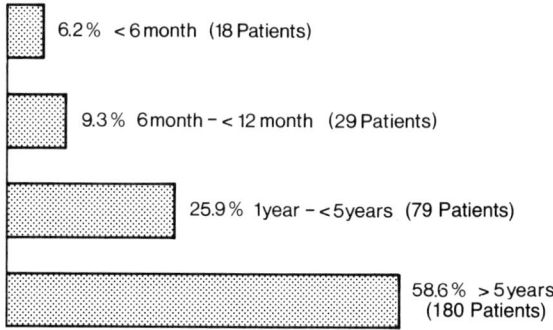

Figure 1. Duration of the pain.

Duration of pain was the variable criterion in our regression analysis. Multiple regression revealed a significant result only in the reporting of bodily complaints, with the strongest variable being "musculo-skeletal complaints" (Table 1). The more people suffer from pain, the more they report bodily complaints, especially symptoms arising from muscles and ligaments. Apart from these results, which fit the hypochondria concept, we found no correlation between duration of pain and other personality traits. The hypothesis postulating this must thus be rejected in the case of our clinical subjects. Only part of our results constituting an "algogenic psychosyndrome" was confirmed. But it does indicate a psychosomatic impact.

Environmental items, such as strain in private and public situations, which were operationalized by the scales "social status," and "social activity" of the BIV, could not be brought into relation with pain duration. Although social disturbances in particular were often reported by those pain patients with long periods of pain, regression analysis did not support this assumption. This is also true for the rest of the personality variables used in this study.

Table 1. Multiple repression with the criterion variable "Duration of Pain." Dependent variables were the scales of the GBB, PDS, and BIV.

	Summary table Duration of Pain			
Variable	Multible R	R Square	Simple R	p
Musculo-Skeletal Complaints	0.26617	0.07085	0.26617	
Cardiac Complaints	0.28936	0.08373	0.03073	
Sum of Physical Complaints	0.33560	0.11263	0.22809	
Indigestion	0.34495	0.11899	0.11351	
Exhaustion	0.34574	0.11954	0.19740	0.05
Denial of Illness	0.11770	0.01385	0.11770	
Depression	0.13157	0.01731	0.08686	
Paranoia	0.13188	0.01739	0.07030	n.s.
Social Status	0.17138	0.02937	0.17138	
Family Situation	0.20756	0.04308	0.15798	
Extraversion	0.23787	0.05658	−0.11173	
Psychophysical Constitution	0.25422	0.06463	0.15271	
Parenting Behavior	0.26058	0.06790	0.10554	
Ego-Strength	0.26437	0.06989	0.15555	
Neurotizism	0.26973	0.07275	0.08346	
Social Activity	0.27251	0.07426	0.14433	n.s.

In contrast to our assumptions, in most scales of the personality test pain patients had no higher scores than people without pain (Figure 2). Our results were only significant for those scales describing social situations, both public and private. This indicates a high portion of strain triggered by pain. The scale "psychophysical constitution" also expresses a high disposition to somatic disturbances, low coping capabilities in stress situations, and a general physiologi-

Psychological Profiles of Chronic Pain Patients 155

cal instability. Figure 2 shows the results of all scales for the four pain types. According to these results, pain patients feel very strained by their illness—independent of pain duration. It has a very negative effect in their social environment, such as in their marriage, profession, and social life.

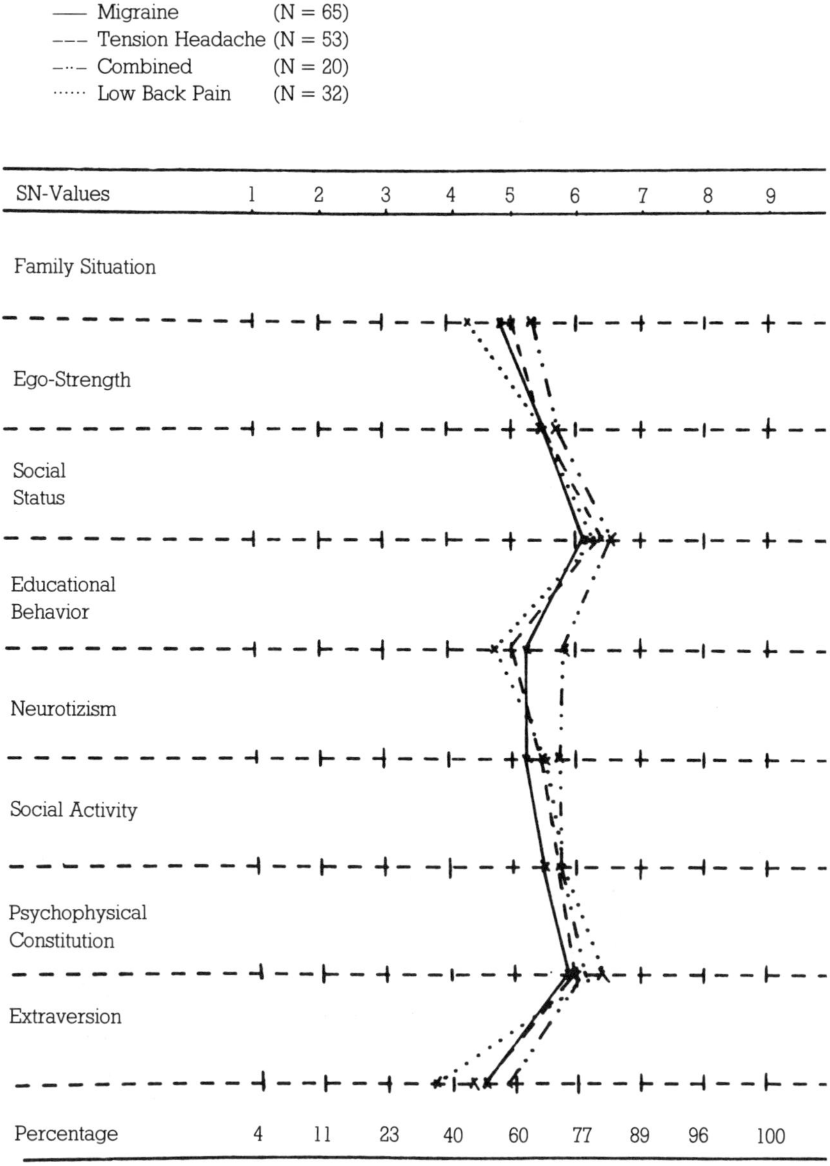

```
——— Migraine          (N = 65)
- - - Tension Headache (N = 53)
-··- Combined          (N = 20)
····· Low Back Pain    (N = 32)
```

| SN-Values | 1 | 2 | 3 | 4 | 5 | 6 | 7 | 8 | 9 |

Family Situation

Ego-Strength

Social Status

Educational Behavior

Neurotizism

Social Activity

Psychophysical Constitution

Extraversion

| Percentage | 4 | 11 | 23 | 40 | 60 | 77 | 89 | 96 | 100 |

Figure 2. Profiles of pain types. Personality scales (BIV).

In Table 2, no differences between the four diagnostic groups can be shown. Neither between all groups, between the individual headache groups, nor between headache sufferers and low back pain patients could we find any significant differences. There is only a trend in our data, migraine patients being least neurotic, patients with tension headache somewhat more so, followed by patients with combined headache.

Table 2. Personality scales (F-values). Analysis of variance (F-values)
— between the different types of pain,
— between the headache types,
— between headache and low back pain patients.

Biographical Inventary	Types of pain		
	all types of pain	headache types	headache vs. low back pain
	p	p	p
Family Situation	0.45	0.68	0.11
Ego-Strength	0.9	0.81	0.83
Social Status	0.7	0.61	0.89
Parenting Behavior	0.39	0.2	0.44
Neurotizism	0.7	0.59	0.71
Social Acitivty	0.28	0.65	0.71
Psychophysical Constitution	0.6	0.67	0.28
Extraversion	0.26	0.45	0.15

The results gained from our "somatic complaints test" confirm that pain patients suffer from many bodily symptoms, particularly from "exhaustion." This is valid for the four pain groups, all of which had significantly higher scores on this scale than their "normal" counterparts, as shown in normative data (Figure 3).

Between the individual headache groups, the variable "indigestion" was significantly different: Migraine patients had the least, patients with combined headches the most complaints on this scale. As is indicated by the mean values, we found a significant difference between headache patients and low back pain patients ($p = 0.03$). Patients with low back pain reported less bodily complaints. On the subscales "exhaustion" and "muskulo-skeletal complaints," these pain groups were strongest apart from each other (Table 3).

All in all, patients with low back pain complained less than the other pain groups. No marked differences between their test scores and normative data

Psychological Profiles of Chronic Pain Patients

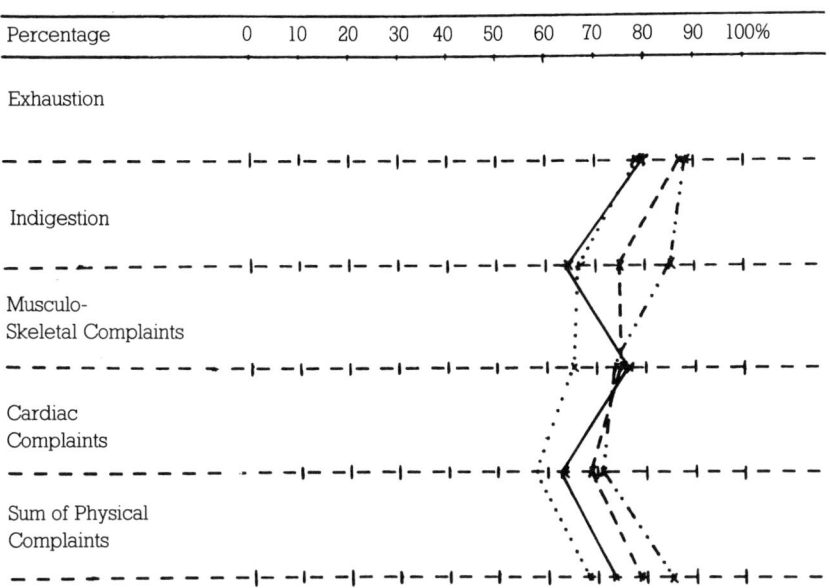

Figure 3. Profiles of pain types. Physical complaints (GBB).

were found. We therefore have to reject our hypothesis regarding the difference between pain groups. Measurements of bodily complaints enable us to differentiate between headache patients and low back pain patients.

Data from the third test, the *Paranoid-Depression Scale* (PDS) indicate that all pain patients had a high depression score, being significantly above normal values (Figure 4). The four pain groups seem to react in an uniform manner. Chronic pain and depression is alike. This is not the case with the paranoia scale. Here, we found normal values in the vascular headache group, followed by patients with low back pain. Patients with combined headaches had the highest values (Table 4). Analysis of variance showed this finding to be significant, stressing the marked difference between patients with migraine headache and patients with combined headaches in this scale. A comparision of the headache groups with the low back pain group did not differentiate the groups on the paranoia scale. The scale "illness denial" proved to be clinically modest within as well as between the different pain groups. A striking feature is the large distribution of this scale.

Table 3. Physical complaints. Analysis of variance (F-values):

- between the different types of pain,
- between the headache types,
- between headache and low back pain patients.

Gießen Symptom Assessment	Types of pain		
	all types of pain	headache types	headache vs. low back pain
	p	p	p
Exhaustion	0.06	0.06	0.045*
Indigestion	0.008**	0.008**	0.15
Musculo-Skeletal Complaints	0.11	0.73	0.008**
Cardiac Complaints	0.17	0.42	0.063
Sum of Physical Complaints	0.02*	0.056	0.03*

* = $p < 0.05$
** = $p < 0.01$

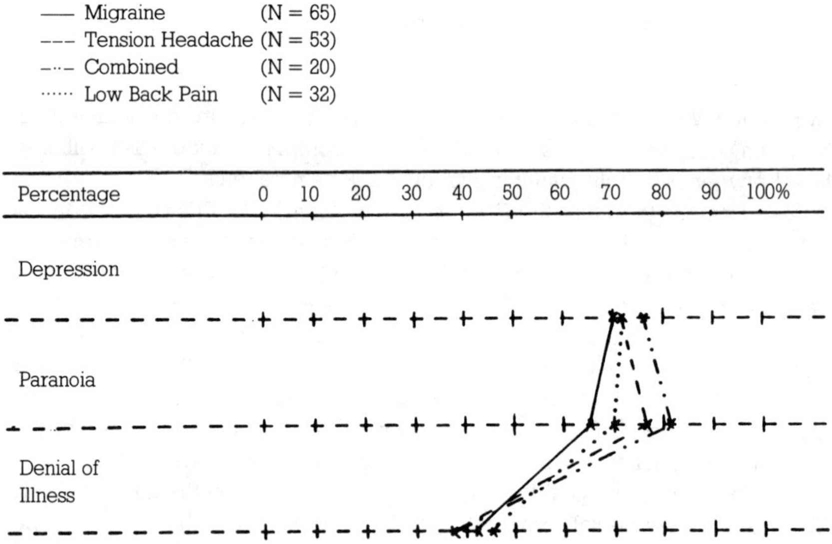

―― Migraine (N = 65)
--- Tension Headache (N = 53)
―·― Combined (N = 20)
······ Low Back Pain (N = 32)

Figure 4. Profiles of pain types. The Paranoid-Depression Scale (PD-S).

Psychological Profiles of Chronic Pain Patients 159

Table 4. The Paranoid-Depression Scale. Analysis of variance (F-values):

- between the different types of pain,
- between the headache types,
- between headache and low back pain patients.

Paranoid-Depression Scale	Types of pain		
	all types of pain	headache types	headache vs. low back pain
	p	p	p
Depression	0.8	0.55	0.88
Paranoia	0.09	0.03	0.65
Denial of illness	0.67	0.64	0.41

* = p < 0.05
** = p < 0.01

We expected gender differences concerning the reporting of somatic complaints. Out of 170 headache and back pain patients, 119 were women, 51 men (Figure 5).

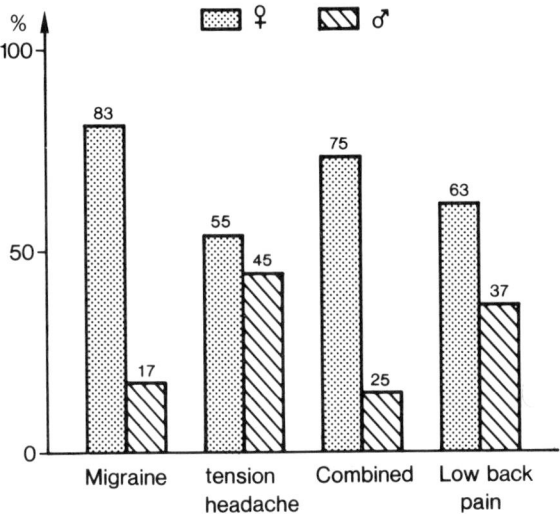

Figure 5. Gender differences in the different pain groups.

Table 5. Multivariate analysis of variance; gender differences by headache and low back pain patients; means and standard deviations in %; F-values.

Gießen Symptom Assessment		Pain Patients				Gender Differences
		males		females		p
		headache	back pain	low ache	hoed- back pain	low
Exhaustion	x	89.9	89.5	82.4	66.4	0.0007**
	s	11.0	7.0	20.4	33.0	
Indigestion	x	78.5	72.4	69.8	58.9	0.054
	s	20.5	23.9	25.8	33.1	
Musculo-Skeletal Complaints	x	77.1	61.0	75.8	64.7	0.8
	s	21.6	21.6	21.1	28.9	
Cardiac Complaints	x	69.6	60.3	67.1	57.1	0.59
	s	19.8	28.5	22.7	32.4	
Sum of Physical Complaints	x	83.0	75.8	75.5	61.4	0.02*
		15.8 19.6	21.8	34.2		

* $p < 0.05$
** $p < 0.01$

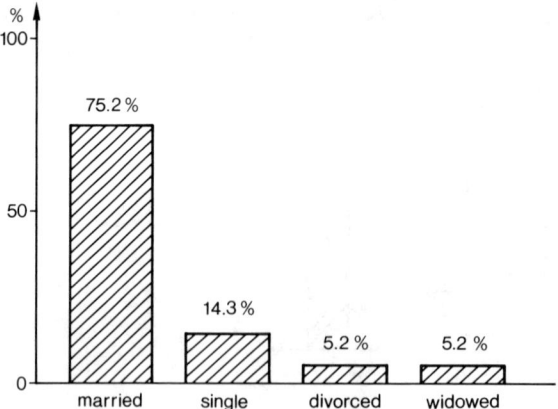

Figure 6. Family status of all pain patients (N = 307).

In our population, four times more women than men suffered from vascular headache. There were only 10% less men with the diagnosis of tension headache. The distribution of gender with combined headache is comparable too with vascular headache. In contrast to this finding, 50% more women than men suffered from backache.

Our hypothesis that women report more bodily complaints, and are thus more psychosomatically disturbed, could not be verified. Taking the sum of complaints made by pain patients, whether complaining of headache or backache, men reported significantly *more* bodily complaints than women (Table 5). The greatest gender difference was in the scale "exhaustion," where male patients complain highly significantly more often than females ($p < 0.01$).

Is the risk of becoming ill connected to family status? Our hypothesis postulated that we would find more singles among pain patients because of a destabilizing social environment, the lack of social support being a health risk factor. Figure 6 shows the family status of 307 patients. 231 (75%) were married, 76 (25%) single, divorced, or widowed. These figures correspond to the general population of West Germany, according to the statistical yearbook of 1987. These results give no indication of an additional health risk or the maintenance of chronic pain being effected by family status.

Discussion

Our results can be summarized as follows: The presence of a pain-induced psychological disorders caused and maintained by the chronification of pain has little support from our data. Multiple regression analysis revealed only that the longer pain exists, the greater the number of somatic complaints reported. This explains only 12% of the variance, but it does indicates the relevance of using symptom-reporting scales in psychosomatic research. More than all other psychological scales, a psychosomatic basis for chronic pain behavior is demonstrated by this subjective measurement.

Other personality traits, such as the "conversion-V" or the so-called "neurotic triad," were not associated with the duration of pain when classified into four periods: up to 1/2 year, 1/2 year to 1 year, 1 to 5 years, and more than 5 years.

The degree of pain reported was found to be associated with stress within the family during leisure and at work. But even these significant findings did not correlate with the duration of pain.

Apart from this aspect, we found that pain patients report significantly more bodily complaints in the scale "psychophysical constitution" (BIV) and in the scales of the *Gießen Symptom Assessment,* which again indicates the psychosomatic impact on pain behavior. These patients were also found to suffer from a marked depression.

Generally, we were able to confirm the presence of a so-called "neurotic triad" (Kudrow & Sutkus, 1979; Andrasik et al., 1982; Sternbach, 1983; Franz et al.,

1986), i.e., the reporting of many somatic complaints (hypochondriosis) in the GBB and the scale "psychophysical constitution" of the BIV. Both scales cover the aspects of "hysteria" as defined in *MMPI*. We also found high depression scores as assessed by the PDS.

The extremly high score for "exhaustion" found in all types of pain patients is in agreement with the findings of Andrasik et al. (1982). In their *MMPI* data these authors observed marked higher scores for psychasthenia when compared with samples drawn from the normal healthy population.

Comparison of the four groups of pain patients reveals slight variations: Those patients with backache had the lowest number of somatic complaints. Only this aspect was significantly different in the low back pain as compared to the headache groups. Murray (1982) commented on the difficulty of distinguishing between organic and psychogenic back pain when using the *MMPI*—indeed, the normality of these patients on psychological evaluation of personality traits and somatic complaints indicates a weakness in this test. That these patients are different from the normal population is shown by the results of Turk and Flor (1984), who described an increase in the EMG activity of the paravertebral musculature when feelings of conflict were provoked. Headache patients have also been found to have higher EMG activity in the musculature of the head and neck (Traue, Bischoff, & Zenz, 1986; Bischoff, Zenz, & Traue, 1986). Social stress led to an increase in muscle activity in these patients which was slower to return to normal resting levels than in healthy volunteers. These results primarily described the psychophysiological mechanisms of headache and low back pain, and can be most frequently elicited in conditions of social stress, whether in the laboratory or in everyday life.

A completely unexpected result of this study was that male chronic pain patients complain significantly more than their female counterparts. This was the case in both the headache and backache groups. This difference may arise because it is pain that forces a previously healthy man to observe his own body, whereas women normally learn to do this without previously having been ill (Mechanic, 1980). Concern over the cause of the complaint may sensitize a man for the first time in this dimension and indirectly lead to a more affect-laden, appellative description.

Not only the above, also a further result of this study does not fit with the current theories: Maritial status, when taken as a measure of social support, or loneliness and depression as compared to support and solidarity, was not found to be correlated in any way with the duration of the pain problem. It may well be that the categories used were too imprecise to enable any sort of prediction to be made, because the social support system may be very defective within an apparently functioning family unit and a vice versa.

Some aspects of social support are assessed by the BIV test, which records social and sexual activity. The former score includes questions describing the patient's capability to form and maintain contacts as well as to communicate with others. The summation of these aspects, which we define as the social situation, was described as being very unsatisfactory by all pain patients. Because we were not able to identify a pain-induced disorder, these results indicate that people coping with chronic pain are in social difficulty. This test score covers other important aspects; however, a greater number of unpleasent life events was found to have occurred in these pain patients. The failure to identify a pain-induced disorder does not mean that chronic pain does not have a negative effect on psychological well-being and behavior. Learning processes leading to better pain coping may suppress a pain-induced disorder. On the other hand, the duration of a chronic pain experience per se does not, apart from the number of somatic symptoms reported, appear to be associated with alterations in psychological well-being.

It may well also be the case that certain types of coping behavior, whether active or passive, modify the development of this disorder (Brown & Nicassio, 1987). Despite the fact that these evalutations revealed no definitive characteristics of chronic pain patients, it would be unwise to refrain from all attempts at obtaining this type of data. In the individual case, the information gained is often of considerable value in further management. In our experience a behavioral analysis including medical, experimental (behavioral testing), and psychosocial components, including psychological testing, should be carried out on all patients presenting with chronic pain.

References

Andrasik, F., Blanchard, E.B., Arena, J.G., Teders, S.J., Teevan, R.C., & Radichak, L.D. (1982). Psychological functioning in headache sufferers. *Psychosomatic Medicine, 44*(2), 171—182.
Bell, N.W., Abramowitz, S.J., Folkins, C.H., Spensley, J., & Hutchinson, G.L. (1983). Biofeedback, brief psychotherapy and tension headache. *Headache, 23,* 162—173.
Beyme, F. (1976), Die Psychosomatik der Kranken mit Migräne und Kopfschmerz. In A. Jores (Ed.), *Praktische Psychosomatik* (pp. 239—255). Bern: Hans Huber.
Bischoff, C., Zenz, H., & Traue, H.C. (1986). Primärer Kopfschmerz. In T. v. Uexküll (Ed.), *Lehrbuch der Psychosomatischen Medizin (pp. 565—582).* München: Urban & Schwarzenberg.
Blaszcynski, A.P. (1984). Personality factors in classical migraine and tension headache. *Headache, 24,* 238—244.
Blanchard, E.B., Andrasik, F., & Arena, J.G. (1984). Personality and chronic headache. In B.A. Maher & W.B. Maher (Eds.), *Progress in experimental personality research, Vol. 13* (pp. 303—364). New York: Academic Press.
Brähler, E., & Scheer, J.W. (1983). *Der Gießener Beschwerdebogen.* Bern: Hans Huber.
Brown, K.G., & Nicassio, P.M. (1987). Development of questionnaire for the assessment of active and passive coping strategies in chronic pain patients. *Pain, 31,* 53—64.
Daalsgaard-Nielsen, T. (1965). Migraine and heredity. *Acta Neurol. Scand., 41,* 287.
Flor, H., & Turk, D.C. (1984). Etiological theories and treatments for chronic back pain. I. Somatic models and interventions. *Pain, 19,* 105—121.
Franz, C., Paul, R., Bautz, M., Choroba, B., & Hildebrandt, J. (1986). Psychosomatic aspects of chronic pain: A new way of description based on MMPI item analysis. *Pain, 26,* 33—43.
Friedman, A.P. (1979). Nature of headache. *Headache, 19,* 163—167.

Geißler, P. (1980). Versagen am eigenen Wertmaßstab als spezifische Konfliktsituation bei Migränepatienten. *Zeitschrift für psychosomatische Medizin, 26,* 40—46.
Haas, J.P. (1985). Die Migräne im Spiegel psychodynamischer Forschungsbeiträge. *Zeitschrift für psychosomatische Medizin, 31,* 14—24.
Hanvik, L.J. (1951). MMPI profiles in patients with low back pain. *Journal of Consulting Psychology, 15,* 350—353.
Harper, R.G., & Heyer, J.C. (1978). Psychological correlates of frontalis EMG in tension headache. *Headache, 18,* 215—218.
Holroyd, K.A., & Andrasik, F. (1978). Coping and the self control of chronic tension headache. *Journal of Consulting and Clinical Psychology, 46,* 1036—1045.
Jäger, R., Lischer, S., Münster, B., & Ritz, B. (1976). *Biographisches Inventar zur Diagnose von Verhaltensstörungen (BIV).* Göttingen: Hogrefe.
Knapp, T.W. (1983). *Migräne I. Symptomatologie und Ätiologie.* Weinheim, Basel: Beltz.
Köhler, Th., Kraus, J., & Vanselow, B. (1987). Die "Migränepersönlichkeit"—mehr als ein Mythos? *Psychotherapie und Medizinische Psychologie, 37,* 170—174.
Kröner, B. (1982). Untersuchung zur Persönlichkeitsstruktur von Patienten mit unterschiedlichen Kopfschmerzsyndromen. *Diagnostica, 28,* 168—184.
Kudrow, L., & Sutkus, B.J. (1979). MMPI pattern specificity in primary headache disorders. *Headache, 19,* 18—24.
Larbig, W. (1982). *Schmerz. Grundlagen—Forschung—Therapie.* Stuttgart: Kohlhammer.
Leavitt, F., & Sweet, J.J. (1986). Characteristics and frequency of malingering among patients with low back pain. *Pain, 25,* 357—364.
Love, A.W., & Peck, C.L. (1987). The MMPI and psychological factors in chronic low back pain: A review. *Pain, 28,* 1—12.
McGill, J.C.; Lawlis, G.F., Selby, D., Mooney, V., & McCoy, C.E. (1983). The relationship of MMPI profile clusters to pain behaviors. *Journal of Behavior Medicine, 6,* 77—92.
Mechanic, D. (1980). The experience and reporting of common physical complaints. *Journal of Health and Social Behaviour, 21,* 146—155.
Murray, J.B. (1982). Psycholocial aspects of low back pain. *Psychological Report, 50,* 343—351.
Pennebaker, J.W. (1982). *The psychology of physical symptoms.* New York: Springer.
Peters, U.H. (1983). *Die erfolgreiche Therapie des chronischen Kopfschmerzes.* Erlangen: Perimed Fachbuch-Verlagsgesellschaft.
Philips, C. (1976). Headache and personality. *Journal of Psychosoamtic Research, 20,* 535—542.
Rosen, J.C., Frymoyer, J.W., & Clements, J.H. (1980). A further look at validity of the MMPI with low back patients. *Journal of Psychosomatic Research, 36,* 994—999.
Selby, G., & Lance, J.W. (1960). Observations on 500 cases of migraine and allied vascular headache. *Journal of Neurology, Neurosurgery and Psychiatry, 23,* 23.
Statistisches Jahrbuch (1987). Stuttgart: Kohlhammer.
Sterling, P., & Eyer, J.C. (1981). Biological basis of stressrelated mortality. *Social Science and Medicine, 15,* 3-42.
Sternbach, R.A. (1983). *Pain-patients: Traits and treatment.* New York: Academic Press.
Sternbach, R.A. (1983). *Schmerzpatienten. Krankheitsursachen und Behandlung.* Heidelberg: Verlag für Medizin Dr. E. Fischer.
Traue, H.C., Gottwald, A., Henderson, P.R., & Bakal, D.A. (1985). Nonverbal expressiveness and EMG activity in tension headache sufferers and controls. *Journal of Psychosomatic Research, 29,* 4, 375—381.
Traue, H.C., Bischoff, C., & Zenz, H. (1986). Sozialer Streß, Muskelspannung und Spannungskopfschmerz. *Zeitschrift für Klinische Psychologie, 15,* 57—70.

Turk, D.C., & Flor, H. (1984). Etiological theories and treatments for chronic back pain. II. Psychological models and interventions. *Pain, 19,* 209—233.
Turk, C.D., & Rudy, Th.E. (1987). Towards a comprehensive assessment of chronic pain patients. *Behaviour Research and Therapy, 25, 4,* 237—249.
Weatherhead, A.D. (1980). Headache associated with psychiatric disorders: Classification and etiology. *Psychosomatics, 21,* 832—840.
Wolff, H.G. (1937). Personality features and reactions of subjects with migraine. *Arch. Neurol. Psych., 37,* 895—918.
v. Zerssen, D., & Köhler, D.M. (1976). *Paranoid-Depressivitäts-Skala.* Weinheim: Beltz.

Motivational and Volitional Characteristics of Patients with a Prolapsed Intervertebral Disk and of Depressed Patients

Roland Straub, Christfried Mayer, Walter Fröscher

In honor of Prof. Dr. G. Hole on his 60th birthday

Motivational and volitional states play a fundamental part in the etiology, perception and processing of back pain. To date, studies have stressed the influence of affective and cognitive components, even though clinical descriptions have revealed differences in the motivation towards action. Active, restless persons for whom success and recognition represents a challenge are distinguished from rather unconfident persons, guided by failure and often depressed, whose main topic is overtaxation and who tend to have more frequent chronic back pain.

We tested a group of 22 patients with acute prolapsed intervertebral disk matched for age and sex with a group of healthy subjects and a group of depressed patients using a questionnaire based on the theory of motivation. We wanted to see whether these clinical characteristics would also be revealed here. We also did a multidimensional analysis. The prolapsed disk patients who were clearly action-oriented had a strikingly positive way of describing themselves as well as a remarkable discrepancy between the reported and physiologically registered level of activation in the EDA. This group differed clearly from the control group in this area as well as in its orientation to norms.

It is now a well-known fact that in painful degenerative spine illnesses neither degeneration nor pain can be explained by organic processes and damage alone. Research into back pain has given special emphasis to the problem of "chronic back pain." Patients with chronic back pain can, allegedly, be described as individuals with a pain-prone personality.

From a nosological point of view, this "pain-prone personality" has mainly been considered to be a particular variant of the depressive syndrome or of masked depression (see, e.g., Forrest & Wolkind, 1974; Maruta, Swanson, & Swanson, 1976; Blumer & Heilbronn, 1982; Hasenbring & Ahrens, 1987).

Roy, Thomas, and Matas (1984), however, warn against putting chronic pain too quickly into the category of clinical depression, in spite of unquestionable

---

This research was supported in part by the DFG (German Research Society) and carried out by the Research Group "Clinical Psychophysiology" of the Depression Treatment and Research Ward in cooperation with the Department of Neurology (Head: Prof. Dr. W. Fröscher), both part of the State Mental Hospital Weissenau, Department of Psychiatry I (Head: Prof. Dr. G. Hole), University of Ulm, Ravensburg-Weissenau, West Germany. Translated by Jennifer Hartog. Our thanks to Sylvia Hoffmann and Peter Lauwasser for helping us with the statistical analyses.

similarities, for example, on the psychosocial and biochemical level, as the existing studies have many methodological and diagnostic weaknesses.

The diagnosis "masked depression" is of little nosologic clarity; it is not usually considered to be a category of its own but rather a handy didactic trick for medical training (Pöldinger, 1982, 60). It also justifies the treatment of such cases with antidepressant medication, thereby neglecting the need for differential diagnosis of the intrapsychic processes at work.

These intrapsychic processes with their emotional, cognitive, motivational, and volitional components, however, modulate the perception and processing of pain considerably. Only when we know exactly how these subsystems are structured and interact will we be able to differentiate and improve diagnostic and therapeutic decisions.

In this paper we concentrate on the influence of motivational components in back pain, as we think that their role in the etiology and persistence of back pain has not been explored enough to date in experimental work. We make our point with a comparative study of patients with an acutely prolapsed intervertebral disk, depressive inpatients, and healthy controls.

Clinical Characterization of the Personality Traits of Patients with Back Pain

Much of the research done into back pain still draws on psychoanalytical and psychosomatic approaches to explain its etiology. These approaches are mostly based on Reich (1970) or Alexander (1950). New studies usually take these psychodynamic relations for granted and merely supplement them with differentiated descriptions of neuropsychological and physiological aspects (Turk & Flor, 1984).

Though it remains debatable whether a "slipped disk personality" really exists, clinicians continue to describe such a personality. Such persons are characterized as being active, restless, and innerly driven; they are said to be in "high spirits" and to idealize themselves, to swoop from omnipotence to helplessness, and to depend extremely on recognition and praise (for a summary, see Kütemeyer & Schultz, 1986).

Apart from these persons, there is a second smaller subgroup of patients who suffer from chronic back pain, especially in the lumbar region. Increased depressive mood is often ascribed to them, and they often observe their own physical symptoms with anxiety. Ahrens (1986) describes these patients as being rigid and self-controlled, as giving the impression they are always pulling themselves together, and as developing a sort of tense activism. This attitude is also referred to as the "grin and bear it" syndrome.

If we compare both descriptions, we notice the partly contrary psychophysical characteristics: patients belonging to the group of persons with the "slipped disk personality" seem to be anything but depressed—quite contrary to the subgroup of patients with "low back pain personality."

The first group of patients causes little trouble in the hospital and wants to be discharged rapidly because of its extreme activeness; the patients of the second group are often in a depressed mood and suffer from chronic pain. As it is often difficult to identify this problem group, a special screening method was developed early on (cf., e.g., Hanvik, 1951).

Typical Motivational Characteristics Concerning Achievement in Back Pain Patients

A salient characteristic of back pain patients is their pronounced focus on achievement—be it success or failure. With respect to achievement, we can distinguish two subgroups of back pain patients. In one subgroup, patients show an orientation toward achievement (in order to gain praise and success) and especially action, combined with high physical and cognitive stress. The second subgroup is characterized by overtaxation combined with psychophysical lability, problems of self-esteem, and orientation toward failure (Kröber, 1985). Especially this latter group causes clinicians considerable problems as these patients have a tendency to develop chronic pain syndromes. Further, this group has similar autonomous and psychological complaints to those which are typical of depressed patients (cf., e.g., Hasenbring & Ahrens, 1987).

Since Melzack and Wall's multi-modal gate control theory (1965), it has been an accepted fact that affective, cognitive, and motivational factors contribute to the development and persistence of pain. Nevertheless, only the affective and especially the cognitive components in the processing of and coping with pain have been discussed and analyzed up to now (cf., e.g., Turk & Meichenbaum, 1983; Flor 1987).

In the diathesis-stress model proposed by Flor (1984), which is at the center of scientific discussion at the moment, the idea of overtaxation is mentioned; the motivational and volitional persisting states, however, which are closely linked to this overtaxation, are not dealt with in depth.

On the basis of experimental data, Flor, Turk, and Birbaumer (1985) pointed out that abnormally high muscle tension during subjectively stressing situations were found only among the so-called chronic back pain patients and not in control groups with or without pain. The EMG parameter correlated with depression (*Beck Depression Inventory*, Beck et al., 1961) as well as with negative cognitive and emotional assessment of pain (*Pain Experience Scale*, Turk 1981). This study stresses, once again, the orientation of this group of patients toward failure, but does not analyze the achievement motive as an etiological factor either.

The Role of Motivation in the Genesis of Back Pain

Besides the cognitive and emotional subsystems, the motivational subsystem, which determines largely choice, duration, and strain of action as well as wishes, values, and intentions, deserves more attention: We think that motivational and volitional processes are closely connected to action. They lead more quickly to specific motoric tension patterns than cognitive processes.

Following the ideas of Kuhl (1983a, 1984; Kuhl & Helle, 1986), we expect differences in information processing, depending on whether the emphasis is on the cognitive, emotional, or motivational subsystems. Motivational states are especially characterized by the fact that they are longer lasting and more related to goal-states of the organism in its interaction with the environment than, for instance, cognitive elements are. Furthermore, they have a stronger impact on the stimulation and impairment of action.

We want to relate the obvious and relatively persistent affective-motivational and volitional characteristics, which determine human action and which always develop within a social context, to the genesis of back pain. For this purpose, we used Kuhl's (1983a) model of action motivation:

This model distinguishes between two types of persons: action-oriented and state-oriented persons. According to Kuhl (1984) and Kuhl and Helle (1986), state-orientation is an essential pre-condition for depression. To date, however, there have been no differential statements as to whether pronounced action-orientation also favors psychological disorders.

State-oriented persons typically exhibit fear of failure. This indicates their striving for social acceptance. They react emotionally very strongly to failure and tend to stay stuck in these "negative experiences," which, in turn, block them for new experiences and actions. The experience of repeated failure leads to a motivational state characterized by dwelling over the last failure and the negative emotions it engenders, instead of re-orientating attention in a way which is more adapted to the situation, toward present and future action. In contrast, action-oriented persons seem to be decidedly more oriented toward success. They quickly turn toward new goals when the aims they were striving for prove to be unrealistic.

There are salient similarities between the two groups of back pain patients just characterized and described in psychoanalytic literature and the motivational types of Kuhl. Tension in the back and degenerative processes favoring the probability of a disk prolapsing are, in the case of a state-oriented person, more likely to be caused by anxiety, problems of self-esteem, and expectations of failure as well as by the accompanying state of being cognitively and emotionally overtaxed.

Because of the perseverance of state-oriented cognitions in the working memory, these tensions persist in a maladapted way and go along with generally increased physical and behavioral arousal.

On the other hand, we expect that clearly action-oriented persons should show such motoric tension patterns rather too often, as the continuous striving toward action goals, in the external world, should impair self-perception during action.

Negative emotions that block action and concomitant cognitive and somatic symptoms are more often suppressed. Because of the strong emphasis on goals, we presume that the patients would often show deficits in perceiving the limits of stress in the back.

Questions and Hypotheses

With the following study we tried to answer two questions:

- Is it possible to distinguish back patients from others by means of Kuhl's *HAKEMP* questionnaire (Action-Control Scale), which is founded on the theory of motivation?
- Can a multidimensional analysis of the different behavioral levels and particularly the motivational aspects reveal the personality characteristics described in the literature as being typical of back pain patients, and thus discriminate them from other groups?

In order to answer these questions, we matched depressed patients and healthy controls for age and sex with non-selected inpatients suffering from acute disk trouble. We expect the depressed patients, in comparison with the healthy controls, to show distinct state-orientation. As for the prolapsed disk patients, our prediction depends on the history of the pain. We also expect that patients without chronic pain and who can be characterized as having a "slipped disk personality" would show marked action-orientation in the *HAKEMP*, just as we expect the patients with chronic back pain to be rather more state-oriented. In addition we want to test whether the groups reveal typical and distinct profiles by means of a multidimensional analysis containing several self-assessment questionnaires pertaining to achievement, affective and motivational aspects of personality as well as psychophysiological and autonomous variables.

We further expect the prolapsed disk patients—contrary to the depressed patients—to show a positive self-description and pronounced action-orientation with signs of increased behavioral activity.

Method

Subjects

We included in our sample a total of 22 women with the primary diagnosis ICD-9:722.1 who had been admitted to the Department of Neurology either for a diagnosis and/or treatment because of acute disk complaints. With the exception of two patients, all the patients had a long history—some as long as 10 years—of degenerative processes of the spine which had received conservative treatment or been operated on. None of the patients, however, presented a clear chronic pain syndrome, nor a primarily depressive syndrome.

The neurological patients were matched according to age and sociodemographic status with patients of the Weissenau Depression Treatment and Research Ward who were suffering either from neurotic depression (ICD-9:300.4) or from lasting depressive reaction (ICD-9:309.1). These diagnoses correspond closest to a "Major Depression" in the DSM III. The patients were selected from a large sample of depressive patients who had already taken part in a routine experiment for another research project. The matched healthy controls were taken from a sample of women who had answered a newspaper advertisement for a stress/strain experiment. This group, however, did not participate in the entire psychophysiological experiment, so that the physiological data in parentheses stem from a non-matched healthy group.

Experimental Conditions and Procedures

In the course of the "routine experiment," data were collected for the following levels of assessment:

The day before the routine experiment, the patients were asked to fill out the *Freiburger Persönlichkeitsinventar-R* (Freiburg Personality Inventory, FPI-R; Fahrenberg, Hampel, & Selg, 1984) and the *HAKEMP* (Action Control Scale; Kuhl, 1985) with its two subscales, the HOM (action orientation after failure) and

Table 1. Measurement tools used in the multi-dimensional analysis.

	psychiatric/neurological diagnoses (ICD-)	
personality	multi-dimentional personality questionnaire concerning strain/stress	FPI-R (Fahrenberg-et al., 1984)
motivational and volitional level	action/state orientation	HAKEMP-questionnaire (Kuhl, 1983a)
affective level	depth of depression	Self-Depression-Scale (Zung, 1965)
	anxiety/fearfulness	State-Trait-anxiety (Laux et al., 1981)
psychophysiological level	activeness, reactiveness	habituation of the OR in the EDA, heartrate;
physical complaints	physical state of health, autonomous symptoms, pain	B−L' (v. Zerssen, 1976)

the HOP (prospective action orientation). High values in the Action Control, HOM and HOP scales indicate action-orientation; low values indicate state-orientation. The control group took all the tests on the same day. Just before the routine test in the psychophysiological laboratory, the subjects had to fill out the Trait Subscale of the *Trait-State-Anxiety Scale* (STAI; Laux, Glanzmann, Schaffner, & Spielberger 1981) and the *Self-Depression Scale* (SDS; Zung, 1965).

First, skin conductance was recorded from the non-dominant hand (on the middle joint of the index and of the middle finger), then the subjects filled out the State Anxiety Subscale of the *STAI* and a complaint list (B-L'; v. Zerssen, 1976).

After the auditory threshold had been determined, the instructions were given for the habituation experiment. Relaxing music was played for 2 minutes, then resting levels were registered over a period of 3 minutes. Thereafter, the habituation experiment started with 10 tones of 1000 Hz, 80 dB, followed by 3 tones of 800 Hz, 80 dB. In all cases, the tone lasted 1 second with an interval between the stimuli of 15 to 25 seconds.

Statistical Analysis

We reduced the data of the various analyses in the same way as in our previous studies concerning state-orientation in the depressive syndrome (Straub & Keller, 1984). All the statistical group comparisons were carried out with the appropriate t-test.

Table 2. Diagnoses and means of the samples of each of the matched groups: P (prolapsed disk patients), C (healthy controls) an D (depressed patients)

	P (n = 22)	C (n = 22)	D (n = 22)	P v C	P v D	C v D
nosological diagnosis ICD-9	722.1		300.4, 309.1 301.4			
age	42.7	39.5	41.1	ns	ns	ns
depression/SDS	32.9	32.6	54.3	ns	.001	.001
HAKEMP (whole)	26.0	22.7	13.3	ns	.001	.001
HOM	12.3	9.8	5.6	ns	.001	.01
HOP	13.7	13.4	7.7	ns	.001	.001

Results

The means and standard deviations for the HOM and HOP subtests and for the total value of the *HAKEMP* as well as age, diagnosis, and depression scores for the matched groups are shown in Table 2.

For the detailed analysis we divided all three groups along the median of the HOM or *HAKEMP* values in the control group. Table 3 reveals that the back pain patients are clearly more action-oriented than the patients in both the other groups, just as the depressed patients are markedly state-oriented.

Table 3. Division along the median of the healthy controls (C) in the *HAKEMP* (whole test) and the HOM subtest; significance levels (chi-square).

		P	C	D	P v C	P v D	D v C
HAKEMP (Md = 23)	Lo	6	11	18	ns	.001	.05
	Ho	16	11	4			
HOM (Md = 9.5)	Lo	4	11	16	.05	.001	ns
	Ho	18	11	5			

Using the multidimensional analysis, the following profiles specific to groups became apparent (Table 4). The depressed patients have clearly increased values ($p < 0.001$) in the depression and anxiety questionnaires, whereas the back pain patients additionally differ from the healthy controls in their low trait anxiety ($p < 0.05$).

If we look at the dimensions of the FPI, the striking point about the back pain patients, compared to the healthy controls, is that, in accordance to the low anxiety level, they describe themselves as being norm-oriented (FPI-R N), emotionally stable, calm, and composed (FPI-R 5), in good spirits and confident (FPI-R 1), having less physical complaints. These differences, which are all statistically significant, correspond to a large extent to the clinical characterization of the "slipped disk personality." On the other hand, we do not find the characteristics of the "chronic back pain patient" such as increased depression, problems of self-esteem and anxiety.

The results on the psychophysiological level seem to contradict the self-descriptions of the back pain patients. These patients show significantly heightened reactivity (hab) and low skin conductance levels with a trend toward increased fluctuations (SFL), i.e., signs of increased psychophysiological activation. They consider themselves, however, to be calm and composed.

The group of depressed patients is, in almost all dimensions, the exact opposite: It differs from both of the other groups on all levels.

Table 4. Comparison of the means (t-test p ≤ .05) of the matched groups P (prolapsed disk patients), C (healthy controls), and D (depressed patients).

		P (n = 18)	C (n = 18)	D (n = 18)	P v C	P v D	C v D
Affective level							
depression symptoms	SDS	32.0 (5.7)	32.7 (7.9)	54.4 (4.3)	ns	.001	.001
anxiety	TRAIT	36.9 (9.0)	37.0 (8.7)	60.6 (9.5)	ns	.001	.001
aggressiveness	FPI-R 6	3.6 (2.1)	5.4 (1.7)	4.8 (1.9)	.05	ns	ns
emotional lability	FPI-R N	3.7 (1.4)	5.6 (2.5)	7.5 (1.3)	.05	.001	.05
physical complaints	FPI-R 8	4.4 (0.6)	5.5 (1.8)	6.4 (1.4)	ns	.001	ns
	BL'	22.1 (7.6)	16.0 (8.1)	38.6 (10.5)	ns	.001	.001
openness/orientation towards socially accepted norms	FPI-R 10	3.8 (1.2)	5.5 (1.7)	5.2 (1.3)	.01	.01	ns
contentedness with life	FPI-R 1	6.8 (1.2)	5.1 (1.9)	2.3 (1.2)	.05	.001	.001
strain/stress	FPI-R 7	4.8 (1.5)	5.3 (2.2)	6.3 (1.5)	ns	.05	ns
Psychophysiological level (reactiveness)							
subjective assessment: inhibition	FPI-R 4	4.5 (1.5)	5.0 (2.1)	6.3 (1.1)	ns	.01	ns
arousal	FPI-R 5	3.4 (1.3)	5.7 (2.0)	6.3 (1.4)	.01	.001	ns
physiological measures: EDA	HAB	7.2 (3.8)	4.4 (3.5)	2.1 (3.6)	.05	.001	ns
	NIV (µS)	3.3 (7.0)	4.6 (9.6)	2.0 (4.6)	ns	.05	.01
	SFL (Ruhe)	13.2 (14.0)	5.4 (7.7)	3.1 (5.0)	ns	.01	ns
ECG	HR	73.3 (9.7)	74.1 (9.6)	86.5 (10.0)	ns	.01	.001

Discussion

The group of back pain patients differs markedly from the healthy controls and the depressed patients. These patients always describe themselves in self-assessment tests concerning behavior in a positive way, or rather in a manner guided by social norms, whereas the depressed patients describe themselves in just the opposite way.

The correspondence to the motivational characteristics underlined in the psychoanalytic studies concerning the psychosomatics of patients with prolapsed intervertebral disk (e.g., Kütemeyer & Schultz, 1986) is obvious. This proves the importance of motivational modulation, which plays an essential role in generating both the cognitive-affective and the actional processes (e.g., Kuhl, 1983c), thereby also playing an essential part in the shaping of pain perception.

The striking thing about the back pain patients is the discrepancy between their excitability, which they subjectively rate as being much lower compared to how the healthy controls and the depressed patients rate themselves, and the registered signs of increased psychophysiological reactivity in the EDA. This could be a sign that these patients have disorders in their self-perception of processes of excitement and of muscular contraction. The beginning of muscular contractions in the back and the pain they cause together with emotional problems are almost completely ignored as the patients' attention is always focusing anew on other action goals. This pressure to be in action is probably caused by the striving for recognition from other/important persons by succeeding and showing themselves in a positive light. If this is so, then motivational modulation plays an essential role in the etiology of back pain, especially in this group.

It would be a very important step to replace the screening methods used to select patients with chronic back pain; methods such as the *MMPI* (Hanvik, 1951) or the *Beck Depression Inventory* recommended by Hasenbring and Ahrens (1987) are hardly backed up by differential psychology. It would seem appropriate to replace them by a multidimensional method founded on the theory of motivation, which could reveal the intrapsychic processes involved in the development of degenerative processes in the different groups.

Referring to the discussion of the "psychosomatics of intervertebral disks" (Ahrens, 1986; Flor, 1984), this would enable the importance of motivational and volitional modulation in the development and persistence of back pain to be set on a broader and more solid foundation in differential psychology concerning the interaction between emotions, cognition and motivation.

Obviously, these first results, which have only a small statistical basis, should be more widely tested. It would be especially important to analyze a group of patients with chronic back pain, which we did not find in our sample. It became clear, however, that motivational particularities could also be shown in the group of patients with intervertebral disk problems, a group that has been termed "non-problematic" by organic medicine until now. And since these persons, who are rather more action-oriented, probably present fewer pain complaints (Kuhl

1984), attention has been mainly focused on the problem group with chronic pain.

These patients, who represent the largest group, are usually quickly discharged from the hospital after conservational or surgical treatment—because of their very activeness. It is less usual for this group to develop chronic pain. A high percentage of these patients, however, continues to have disk problems and to be operated on, which shows the urgent need for psychologically founded preventive measures.

Seen from the angle of prevention, great attention should be paid in the future to studying the part played by differential-psychological, and especially motivational, factors in maintaining behavioral patterns that favor the progressive degeneration of the spine because of overtaxation of the muscular-skeletal system.

References

Ahrens, S. (1986). Chronische Lumbo-Ischialgie: Der Kranke nimmt sich zu scharf an die Kandare. *Ärztliche Praxis, 43,* 1514—1517.
Alexander, F. (1950). *Psychosomatic medicine.* New York: Norton.
Beck, A.T., Ward, C.H., Mendelson, M. et al. (1961). An inventory for measuring depression. *Archives of General Psychiatry, 4,* 561—571.
Blumer, D., & Heilbronn, M. (1982). Chronic pain as a variant of depressive disease. The pain-prone disorder. *Journal of Nervous and Mental Disease, 170,* 381—406.
Dahlstrom, W.G., Welsh, W.S., & Dahlstrom, L.E. (1972). *An MMPI Handbook, Vol. 1, Clinical interpretation.* Minneapolis: University of Minnesota Press.
Fahrenberg, J., Hampel, R., & Selg, H. (1984). *Das Freiburger Persönlichkeitsinventar (FPI-R). 4. revidierte Auflage.* Göttingen: Hogrefe.
Flor, H. (1984). *Empirical evaluation of a diathesis-stress modell of chronic back pain.* Dissertation, University of Tübingen.
Flor, H., Turk, D.C., & Birbaumer, N. (1985). Assessment of stress-related psychophysiological reactions in chronic back pain patients. *Journal of Consulting and Clinical Psychology, 53,* 345—364.
Flor, H. (1987). Die Rolle psychologischer Faktoren bei der Entstehung und Behandlung chronischer Wirbelsäulensyndrome. *Psychotherapie und medizinische Psychologie, 37,* 424—429.
Forrest, A.J., & Wolkind, S.N. (1974). Masked depression in men with low back pain. *Rheumatology and Rehabilitation, 13,* 148—153.
Fordyce, W.E. (1982). A behavioral perspective on chronic pain. *British Journal of Clinical Psychology, 21,* 313—323.
Hanvik, L.J. (1951). MMPI-profiles in patients with low back pain. *Journal of Consulting Psychology, 15,* 350—353.
Hasenbring, M., & Ahrens, S. (1987). Depressivität, Schmerzwahrnehmung und Schmerzerleben bei Patienten mit lumbalem Bandscheibenvorfall. *Zeitschrift für Psychotherapie, Psychosomatik und Medizinische Psychologie, 37,* 149—155.
Kröber, H.-L. (1985). Zur Klinik und Entstehung psychogener Schmerzsyndrome. *Nervenarzt, 56,* 237—244.

Kuhl, J. (1983a). Handlungs- und Lageorientierung: Empirische Untersuchungen zu einem Perseverationsmodell der Handlungskontrolle. In J. Kuhl (Ed.), *Motivation, Konflikt und Handlungskontrolle* (pp. 251—327). Berlin: Springer-Verlag.

Kuhl, J. (1983b). Emotion, Kognition und Motivation: I. Auf dem Wege zu einer systemtheoretischen Betrachtung der Emotionsgenese. *Sprache und Kognition, 2,* 1—27.

Kuhl, J. (1983c). Emotion, Kognition und Motivation. II. Die funktionale Bedeutung der Emotionen für das problemlösende Denken und für das konkrete Handeln. *Sprache und Kognition, 4,* 228—253.

Kuhl, J. (1984). Motivationstheoretische Aspekte der Depressionsgenese: Der Einfluß von Lageorientierung auf Schmerzempfinden, Medikamentenkonsum und Handlungskontrolle. In M. Wolfersdorf, R. Straub & G. Hole (Eds.), *Depressiv Kranke in der Psychiatrischen Klinik* (pp. 411—433). Regensburg: Roderer.

Kuhl, J., & Helle, P. (1986). Motivational and volititional determinants of depression: The degenerated-intention hypothesis. *Journal of Abnormal Psychiatry, 95,* 247—251.

Kütemeyer, M., & Schultz, U. (1986). Psychosomatik des Lumbago-Ischias-Syndroms. In T. von Uexküll (Ed.), *Psychosomatische Medizin* (pp. 835—846). München: Urban & Schwarzenberg.

Laux, L., Glanzmann, P., Schaffner, P., & Spielberger, C. D. (1981). *State-Trait-Angstinventar (STAI).* Weinheim: Beltz.

Maruta, T., Swanson, D.W., & Swanson, W.M. (1976). Pain as a psychiatric symptom: Comparison between low back pain and depression. *Psychosomatics, 17,* 123—127.

Melzack, R., & Wall, P.D. (1965). Pain mechanisms: A new theory. *Science, 150,* 971—979.

Pöldinger, W. (1982). Differenzieren zwischen Psychosomatosen und larvierten Depressionen. *Ärztliche Fortbildung, 18,* 53—64.

Roy, R., Thomas, M., & Matus, M. (1984). Chronic pain and depression: A review. *Comprehensive Psychiatry, 25,* 96—105.

Reich, W. (1970). *Charakteranalyse.* Köln: Kiepenheuer und Witsch.

Straub, R., & Keller, F. (1984). Die Bedeutung der Handlungs- und Lageorientierung bei der differentiellen Betrachtung depressiver Syndrome. In M. Hautzinger & R. Straub (Eds.), *Psychologische Aspekte depressiver Störungen* (pp. 109—133). Regensburg: Roderer.

Turk, D.C., Meichenbaum, D.H., & Genest, M. (1983). *Pain and behavioral medicine: A cognitive-behavioral perspective.* New York: Guilford Press.

Turk, D.C., & Flor, H. (1984). Etiological theories and treatments for chronic back pain. II. Psychological models and interventions. *Pain, 19,* 209—233.

Zerrsen v., D. (1976). *Klinische Selbstbeurteilungsskalen (KSb-S) aus dem Münchner psychiatrischen Informationssystem.* Weinheim: Beltz.

Zung, W.K. (1965). A self rating depression scale. *Archives of General Psychiatry, 12,* 63—70.

SECTION D:
PAIN MANAGEMENT

Biofeedback Applications for Headache

Frank Andrasik

This chapter selectively reviews the vast literature on biofeedback treatment of various headache types. It is an attempt to identify the relevant treatment effects and to show where there are gaps in knowledge. The main topics are treatment efficacy of biofeedback, biofeedback modalities, follow-up studies and pediatric applications of biofeedback procedures.

There is no doubt that biofeedback is an efficient treatment for migraine, tension and mixed headache but not for cluster headache and menstrual migraine. The treatment outcome decreases with age and psychological variables such as depression, anxiety and some MMPI personality variables which are highly correlated with chronicity. The rates of improvement by biofeedback with children and adolescence exceed by far those obtained with adults. This is a strong argument for an early application of biofeedback and related self-regulatory procedures in pain history.

The chapter includes a discussion of treatment mechanisms. Findings from treatment studies are difficult to interpret since the diagnostic procedures with their low reliabilities and the etiological controversies muddle any proper conclusions. In addition, some biofeedback studies have found direction of physiological control to be without relevance for effectiveness thus raising questions about the specificity of biofeedback treatment.

Biofeedback as a treatment for recurrent headache sufferers has shown considerable growth since the initial pioneering work of researchers at the Menninger Clinic, Topeka, KS (Sargent, Green, & Walters, 1972, 1973) and the University of Colorado Medical Center, Denver, Colorado (Budzynski, Stoyva, & Adler, 1970; Budzynski, Stoyva, Adler, & Mullaney, 1973) nearly two decades ago. It seems appropriate at this point to stop and ponder, "What have we learned from the accumulative research to date?" A brief answer is, "Well, we've learned quite a bit; but at the same time, we have much so more to learn." This chapter selectively reviews available biofeedback treatment literature, in an attempt to identify what specifically has been learned from research studies to date and, just as importantly, to pinpoint areas where our knowledge base is lacking and in need of additional research. Space limitations preclude exhaustive coverage. Reference citation is reserved to those studies best illustrating current findings and issues. Specifically addressed are treatment efficacy of biofeedback, alone and in comparison to other treatment modalities (both pharmacological and nonpharmacological); maintenance of treatment effects; indicators of response to

---

Professor & Director of Graduate Studies, Department of Psychology, University of West Florida, 11000 University Parkway, Pensacola, FL 32514-5751; and Neurology and Headache Management Center, 5500 North Davis Highway, Pensacola, FL 32504, USA.

biofeedback therapy, or matching patients to treatments; treatment mechanisms; treatment of children; and alternative treatment delivery approaches.

Treatment Efficacy

Martin (1983) surveyed published behavioral literature from 1972 through 1982 and categorized the research focus of all papers dealing with headache. He found that the vast majority, 75%, dealt with treatment efficacy; a mere 15% were devoted to etiology, and 10% to nosology. The thrust of intervening work, from then until now, continues this preoccupation with the study of clinical efficacy of treatment in isolation of other important considerations. The consequence of continuing the "overexploited strategy of comparing one variant of relaxation or biofeedback training with another" (Martin, 1983, p. 212) has been both good and not so good. Good in the sense that the efficacy of biofeedback is now fairly well established. Comprehensive Task Force Reports, instigated by the Biofeedback Society of America (Andrasik & Blanchard, 1987; Blanchard & Andrasik, 1987), and meta-analytic reviews (Blanchard, Andrasik, Ahles, Teders, & O'Keefe, 1980; Holroyd, 1986; Holroyd & Penzien, 1986) all support the clinical utility of biofeedback therapy (and relaxation as well) for migraine and tension headache. Further, several different medical groups have endorsed biofeedback as an adjunctive treatment procedure for headache (AASH Board of Directors, 1978; American Psychiatric Association, 1980; Diagnostic and Therapeutic Technology Assessment, 1983). Mean improvement rates for biofeedback and relaxation training (the treatment most frequently compared to biofeedback) from three separate meta-analyses are presented in Table 1. Three findings stand out most. First, improvement rates for biofeedback exceed those for no treatment and various control procedures (psychological and pharmacological). Second, treatment effects show some deterioration over time when comparing the most recent meta-analyses to the earlier one. Holroyd and Penzien (1986) compared "early" to more "recent" studies on a number of client dimensions (age, referral source, gender, etc.) and found no reliable way to explain the declining improvement rates. Third, when biofeedback and relaxation are applied separately, improvement levels seem comparable. This latter finding has led some to conclude that biofeedback and relaxation must be interchangeable clinically and operate through similar mechanisms. Others have gone even further, suggesting biofeedback be abandoned in favor of relaxation, which is simpler and less costly to apply. The somewhat increased improvement rate for biofeedback combined with relaxation training argues against such conclusions, as does a recognition of the fallacy of the "patient uniformity myth" which inherently underlies this suggestion.

The problem caused by researchers continuing to succumb to the patient uniformity myth is illustrated in Figure 1. The top panel of Figure 1 reveals the clinical state of affairs where patients and treatments are truly interchangeable. The

Table 1. Average improvement rates from three separate meta-analyses.

Tension Headache	EMGBF	REL	EMG+REL	BFCT	PTCT	MDCT	WTLT
Blanchard et al. (1980)	60.9	59.2	58.8		35.3	34.8	−4.5
Holroyd & Penzien (1986)	46.0	44.6	57.1	15.3			−3.9

Migraine Headache	ATFB	THFB	REL	VMBF	THFB+REL	MDCT	WTLT
Blanchard et al. (1980)	65.1	51.8	52.7			16.5	
Holroyd (1986)		28.1*	44.4	31.3*	57.4		11.0

EMGBF = Electromyographic biofeedback, generally provided from the frontal/forehead muscles.
REL = Relaxation therapy, generally of the muscle tensing and relaxing variety.
BFCT = Biofeedback control procedure, generally false or noncontingent biofeedback.
PTCT = Psychological or pseudotherapy control porocedure.
MDCT = Medical control procedure; results taken from double blind placebo controlled medication trials.
WTLT = Waiting list control procedure.
ATFB = Thermal biofeedback augmented by components of autogenic training, as developed at the Menninger Clinic.
THFB = Thermal biofeedback by itself.
VMBF = Vasomotor biofeedback provided from the temporal artery.

* Initial analyses for treatment of migraine revealed poor results for biofeedback by itself. In subsequent meta-analyses, which controlled for methodological problems inherent in some of the studies, all treatments for migraine, either alone or in combination, were not found to differ statistically and yielded improvement levels of approximately 40%.

lower panel illustrates the case where two different treatments lead to similar rates of improvement on average, but where patients within the respective treatment groups respond differently. The bottom panel illustrates further the case where treatments are interchangeable for a portion of patients (the middle 30%), but not for the remainder. "Horse race" comparisons, pitting biofeedback and other forms of treatment, divorced from rigorous attempts to characterize individual patient responses, will not take us beyond our current empirical base. One way researchers have begun to address the issue of possible differential responsivity of biofeedback and other forms of therapy is adapted from the medical literature—treatment crossover designs. Results from two separate partial crossover evaluations suggest that biofeedback may offer a treatment advantage over relaxation training for certain patients (Blanchard et al., 1982b).

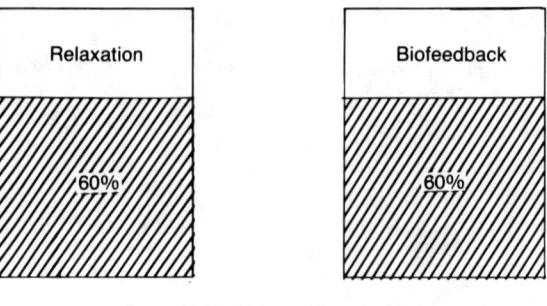

Figure 1. Alternative explanations for equivalent group outcomes.

Same Patient-Types Respond to Each Treatment at Same Level

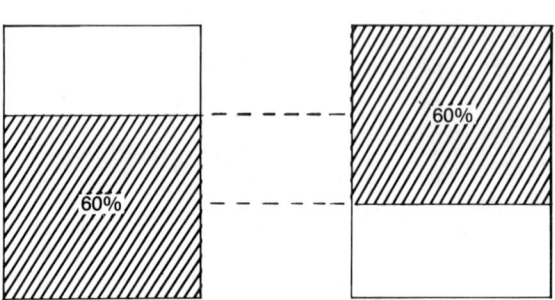

Different Patient-Types Respond to Each Treatment at Same Level

Maintenance of Effects

Although the data base supporting the efficacy of biofeedback is extensive, most of the studies have limited their focus to short-term treatment effects. Nearly two decades after the first successful biofeedback reports appeared in the literature, the grand total of prospective evaluations of the long-term effectiveness of biofeedback (one year and beyond completion of treatment) remains under 10. Available follow-up investigations, assessing patient progress two to four years post-treatment, suggest effects remain fairly robust and durable (Andrasik & Holroyd, 1983; Blanchard, Guarnieri, Andrasik, Neff, & Rodichok, 1987; Ford, Stroebel, Strong, & Szarek, 1983). Caution may be indicated when considering these results, however. Attrition has occurred in all studies, and missing cases have been omitted from analysis, rather than being included and counted as treatment failures (which some may argue is the preferred procedure). This raises the possibility that these favorable long-term outcomes may be positively biased. One study was able to follow a small group of untreated subjects (n = 9) for 3 years, and found headache activity levels remained similar in severity (Andrasik & Holroyd, 1983). Although an admittedly small sample, these findings suggest headache in its untreated state is fairly resilient, and that "regression to the mean" is minimal with this disorder.

Various procedures have been suggested as useful for enhancing maintenance of treatment gains, but few have ever been subjected to controlled evaluation. Most investigators appear to have used the strategy Stokes and Baer (1977) term the "train-and-hope" method. Lynn and Freedman (1979) reviewed the available analog and anecdotal, uncontrolled case study literatures and concluded the following procedures held the greatest promise for helping patients maintain a favorable treatment response over extended time periods: offering booster treatments; fading or gradually increasing the time between treatment appointments; incorporating stimulus control techniques; conducting therapy sessions under stressful or stimulating conditions in order to simulate better the patient's natural environment; varying the stimuli associated with training (using multiple therapists, seeing the patient in several different treatment rooms); or teaching the patient a variety of self-regulation skills to increase the patient's chances of successfully handling all stressful stimuli confronted. Cognitive-behavioral treatments incorporate aspects of the last-mentioned strategy; some biofeedback treatment programs utilize the second strategy as well (fade therapy contact over time).

One follow-up investigation has prospectively studied ways to enhance maintenance. At the end of successful treatment (by either relaxation or relaxation combined with biofeedback) Andrasik, Blanchard, Neff, and Rodichok (1984) randomly assigned patients to one of two prospective follow-up conditions: intensive therapy contact (6 additional or booster treatments spaced over 6 months) or minimal therapist contact (6 brief contacts, of 10—15 minutes duration, again spaced over 6 months). Maintenance rates were identical during the 6 months of additional contact and the 6 months following additional contact. Minimal therapist contact for a brief period after treatment completion may be an efficient, cost-effective way to maintain treatment gains, although this conclusion must remain tentative in that a "no-contact" control group was not included in this study for comparison.

Cognitive Therapy

Cognitive therapies have been attempted with headache patients, but investigations of this procedure are too few in number to be included in the earlier mentioned meta-analyses. Also, most cognitive treatments incorporate aspects of biofeedback or relaxation training, making it impossible to isolate and evaluate the unique contribution of cognitive therapy. Of the three studies evaluating relatively "pure" forms of cognitive therapy, two found equivalent results for it and vasomotor biofeedback with migraine patients (Gerhards, Rojahn, Boxan, Gnade, Petrik, & Florin, 1983; Knapp & Florin, 1981), while the other found stress coping training procedures to be superior to EMG biofeedback for tension headache (Holroyd, Andrasik, & Westbrook, 1977). A 1-year follow-up evaluation for one of the migraine treatment studies (Knapp, 1982) and a 2-year follow-up for the tension headache investigation (Holroyd & Andrasik, 1982) revealed the initial findings were maintained in both cases.

Matching Patients to Treatments

The preoccupation with efficacy research has also been "not so good" because it has siphoned attention away from other important research issues. For example, most of the efficacy trials have failed to incorporate strategies that would allow determination of, to paraphrase a question posed long ago by Kiesler (1966), "what biofeedback treatment works best for what type of patient under what set of circumstances?" When headache patients come to a practitioner's office for biofeedback today, about the best they can be told is, "We know biofeedback works and works well for a majority of patients, but we cannot say with much certainty whether it will work for you, whether another form of treatment might work better, how long treatment might take, etc." The practitioner is left to conclude, "Let's give it a try for a few sessions and then evaluate how things are going." Fortunately, researchers are beginning to address the all important issue of patient-treatment matching.

Age

Increasing age is associated with a decreased response to biofeedback and related self-regulatory treatments such that the odds of a successful treatment response begin to drop out somewhat after age 35—40 (Blanchard et al., 1985b; Diamond & Montrose, 1984; Holroyd & Penzien, 1986). It is difficult to know exactly what to make of this observation. Chronicity is highly correlated with age, but no one has yet attempted to study age in isolation of this variable. Whether this effect is due to biological aging alone thus cannot be determined. Recent research with pediatric headache sufferers reveals enhanced treatment outcomes for children and adolescents. In fact, rates of improvement far exceed those obtained with adult headache sufferers, suggesting children may be especially good candidates for biofeedback and related self-regulatory procedures. More will be said about treatment of pediatric headache in a later section.

Psychological Variables

Elevations on psychological scales measuring anxiety, depression, and related constructs have been found to be predictive of a poor response to self-regulation therapy. Specifically, elevations exceeding the modest value of 8 on the *Beck Depression Inventory* (a finding similar to that reported by Hasenbring in this volume for chronic low back pain patients), moderate elevations on the *State-Trait Anxiety Inventory,* and heightened scores on scales 1, 2, and 3 (primarily) of the *MMPI* have all been found to be correlated with a decreased treatment outcome (Blanchard et al., 1985a; Diamond & Montrose, 1984; Jacob, Turner, Szekely, & Eidelman, 1983; Werder, Sargent, & Coyne, 1981).

A problem for the clinician is deciding how to apply this "predictive" information. When addressing this problem, it is helpful to keep in mind how this information has been collected. In the typical research study, a group of patients is pretested with a comprehensive battery of psychological inventories and then administered a standard treatment package of a set duration. Change in symptom status is then related to initial or pre-test scores via correlational procedures (primarily multiple regression and discriminant function analyses); alternatively, various "cutting scores" are established for the psychological indices to find the ones that best divide patients into successes and failures. Thus, results tell the clinician which patients are unlikely to respond to or may be especially difficult to be helped by the treatment as standardly applied. The test data, unfortunately, do not provide clues as to what else needs to be done for these "at-risk" patients, leaving the clinician with few guides for planning additional treatment options. Further, the stability of individual cutting scores and test predictors must be questioned at the moment, as few findings have been cross-validated to test for "shrinkage effects." Barlow, Hayes, and Nelson (1984) discuss other problems associated with statistical approaches to predicting success and failure.

Refractory Headache Types

Attempts to treat patients diagnosed as having cluster or menstrual migraine by biofeedback and related self-regulation treatments have proven to be largely unsuccessful (Blanchard et al., 1982a; Solbach, Sargent, & Coyne, 1984; Szekely et al., 1986). Still, psychological therapy may be of value to some of these patients in helping them cope better with the distress often resulting from having to endure repeated, intense attacks of these types of headache.

Present research on selecting patients and sequencing treatments remains in the infancy stage. Additional work along the above lines plus incorporation of the "clinical replication" strategies of Barlow, Hayes, and Nelson (1984) is needed.

Biofeedback vs. Medical Treatments

Subjects in virtually all biofeedback treatment studies do not appear to have been weaned from any current medications being taken, nor have they been asked to stabilize their existing medication routines. Thus, nearly all investigations of biofeedback may actually default to studies of biofeedback combined with uncontrolled use of medication. Only recently have researchers attempted to tease out the separate and interactive effects of medication and biofeedback treatment.

For tension headache, EMG biofeedback has been found to be superior to "the most suitable" medical therapy (physical therapy and medication), with results holding through 3 months of follow-up (Bruhn, Olesen, & Melgaard, 1979). In another study (Paiva et al., 1982), diazepam was initially found to be superior to EMG biofeedback; however, at brief follow-up diazepam-treated patients began to reveal pronounced deterioration (a near return of symptoms), while biofeedback-treated subjects now revealed substantial treatment gains. It is unfortunate that longer-term follow-up data were not obtained to see whether the patterns noted at brief follow-up endured.

Two direct comparisons of biofeedback and medication for migraine have been reported, with different outcomes. Sovak, Kunzel, Sternbach, and Dalessio (1981) found propranolol plus occasional analgesics to be similar in effectiveness to biofeedback combined with relaxation, although significantly more attrition occurred for drug therapy. Mathew (1981) compared biofeedback to abortive-plus-analgesic therapy, propranolol, or amitriptyline, and various combinations of drugs and biofeedback, for patients with pure migraine and mixed migraine-muscle contraction. Eight different treatments were compared for each headache type. Just over 800 patients were recruited for the study (which is without a doubt the largest single trial to date); 554 completed all phases of the study. Results are summarized in Table 2. Biofeedback was more effective than abortive/analgesic treatment for both headache types. The three regimens of prophylactic medication (propranolol alone, amitriptyline alone, and the two combined) exceeded biofeedback in most comparisons. Administering biofeedback concurrent with prophylactic medication enhanced effectiveness by an additional 10—20%, supporting the utility of combining medical and biofeedback treatments. For both headache types, the greatest improvement occurred with the combination of some type of prophylactic medication and biofeedback.

Although combining psychological treatment with medication yields enhanced outcome relative to either treatment by itself, research suggests that there may be a minor problem with certain treatment combinations. Jay, Renelli, and Mead (1984) found that propranolol impeded the progress of patients undergoing concurrent thermal biofeedback; curiously, this medication appeared to increase physiological variability. Patients were ultimately able to reach established biofeedback training criteria, but with significantly greater difficulty and increased frustration. Similar interference effects were found for tension

Table 2. Headache improvement as a function of biofeedback and medical treatment (data from Mathew, 1981).

a. Migraine patients

Treatment Condition	Number of Patients Completing Treatment	Percentage of Improvement
(1) Medication Control (Ergotamine + Analgesic)	33	20
(2) Biofeedback	31	35
(3) Amitriptyline	32	42
(4) Amitriptyline + Biofeedback	38	48
(5) Propranolol	38	62
(6) Propranolol + Amitriptyline	38	64
(7) Propranolol + Amitriptyline + Biofeedback	30	73
(8) Propranolol + Biofeedback	33	74

b. Mixed patients

Treatment Condition	Number of Patients Completing Treatment	Percentage of Improvement
(1) Medication Control (Ergotamine + Analgesic)	35	18
(2) Biofeedback	31	48
(3) Propranolol	38	52
(4) Amitriptyline	31	60
(5) Propranolol + Biofeedback	34	62
(6) Amitriptyline + Biofeedback	39	66
(7) Propranolol + Amitriptyline + Biofeedback	36	69
(8) Propranolol + Amitriptyline + Biofeedback	37	76

headache patients receiving EMG biofeedback while simultaneously taking amitriptyline. Informing biofeedback patients about the potential interference effects of these two medications may help minimize frustration and offset lapses in patient motivation.

Medication Rebound Headaches

Recent research suggests that two types of medication commonly prescribed for headache patients, namely, analgesics (Kudrow, 1982; Wörz, 1983) and ergotamine preparations (Ala-Hurula, Myllyla, & Hokkanen, 1982; Saper, 1987; Saper & Jones, 1986; Wörz, 1983), can lead to "rebound" headaches if overused. The term rebound refers both to the worsening of the headache as the medication wears off and to the fact that the patient goes through a marked exacerbation after abrupt discontinuation of the medication (withdrawal-like phenomenon). It is this sequence of symptoms that seduces patients into taking ever-increasing amounts of medication, establishing a vicious cycle. Allowing patients to continue abusively high levels of these medications can compromise an otherwise effective treatment. Kudrow (1982) found a mean improvement rate of only 30% for tension-headache patients treated by amitriptyline when they were permitted to continue their unrestricted use of analgesics. The improvement rate more than doubled (M = 72%) for patients who were given amitriptyline and were concurrently withdrawn from all analgesics. Kudrow found that analgesic withdrawal by itself led to substantial improvement, too (43% symptom reduction). Rapoport, Sheftell, Baskin, and Weeks (1984) reported similar findings. These studies indicate the importance of identifying patients who may be experiencing medication rebound headaches and of helping them to reduce, preferably to eliminate, the medications producing the paradoxical effects on headache.

Mechanisms of Biofeedback Therapy

It has often been said, "Biofeedback is an effective treatment, in search of an explanation." Our knowledge of how biofeedback works with headache patients is poorly understood, as is true in so many areas of treatment. This is due to several reasons. First is the apparent lure or interest in clinical outcome research (recall Martin's, 1983, observations). Second, there is widespread disagreement among researchers about the fundamental nature of the disorder itself. Migraine, for example, is now viewed variously as originating from peripheral vascular abnormalities, biochemical imbalances, neurotransmitter/receptor dysfunction, spreading cortical depression or neuronal suppression, inadequate psychological coping repertoires, and combinations of all the preceding (Saper, 1986). A diagnosis of tension headache is usually made after all other types of headache (functional and organic) have been ruled out (Philips, 1977), making it almost certain that current use of this diagnosis leads to overinclusion. It may very well be that a substantial portion of individuals currently diagnosed as tension headache have no appreciable muscle tension component or are in actuality migraine headaches "transformed" to now resemble tension headache (Mathew, Reuveni, & Perez, 1987). Psychophysiological investigations of migraine and tension headache patients have not been illuminating (Andrasik et al., 1982). Recognition of the likely heterogeneity among a group of patients diagnosed as tension headache has led some researchers to advocate separating this large group of headache sufferers into smaller homogeneous subsets: those with bonafide muscle tension involvement, termed "myogenic" headache (Bischoff & Traue, 1983) and those without, termed, for the moment, "psychogenic head pain" (Haber, Kuczmierczyk, & Adams, 1985). This latter diagnostic category will likely need further refinement, as it too is somewhat of a "grab bag" term. Assessment procedures outlined in Cram (this volume), Haynes (1980), and Schlote (1983) may be helpful in accurately documenting for which headache patients muscle tension is a crucial factor, wherein muscle tension lowering, via biofeedback or related procedures, may be indicated. Conducting assessments and treatments during "dynamic movement" constitute other promising directions (Ahles, King, & Martin, 1984).

Some investigators have gone so far as to conclude that migraine and tension headache are not etiologically distinct. This view places migraine and tension on the same etiological continuum and attributes observed differences in symptom presentation merely to varied degrees of etiologic involvement. This etiologic controversy was discussed at the earlier conference (Bakal, Kaganov, & Demjen, 1983) and continues in full force today (Saper, 1986).

The situation is complicated even further when one realizes potential problems due to diagnostic unreliability. The few studies that have examined diagnostic reliability suggest there may be a serious problem in interpreting the available literature. Interrater reliability coefficients for diagnostic criteria developed and used within a single setting reveal agreement rates of 71% (Turkat, Brantley, Orton, & Adams, 1981) and 86% (Blanchard et al., 1981). Weeks, Baskin, Rapoport, and Sheftell (1984) studied whether diagnostic practices were at all comparable across settings. Fifty different patient histories were prepared and mailed to a large sample of headache specialists employed at various clinics. Participants were asked to make blind diagnoses and to describe the diagnostic system they used and the kind of information they found important in arriving at their decision. Multiple specialists worked in two of the survey settings, which allowed the investigators to calculate rates of diagnostic agreement for professionals employed within a particular setting (and thus permit comparison to the previous two studies already described). Ratings given by individuals working within the same setting revealed perfect agreement in approximately 85% of all cases. Comparison across settings revealed a mean perfect agreement rate of only 52%. Diagnostic agreement rates for four different professional disciplines represented in the study (neurologists, nurses, internists, and psychologists) were strikingly similar and ranged from 53% to 58%. The poor rate of diagnostic agreement across disciplines and settings is viewed as all the more problematic because the majority of raters claimed to be using the same diagnostic system, the one proposed by the Ad Hoc Committee on Classification of Headache (1962)! Findings from these three reliability studies suggest a significant problem with current diagnostic approaches and in interpreting the available literature, in that anywhere from 15% to 48% of cases may be questionably diagnosed. The Ad Hoc Committee of the International Headache Society (1987) has just proposed a new set of diagnostic criteria, which better articulates inclusion and exclusion criteria. However, no reliability field studies have been reported for this new system. In the face of these basic etiologic and diagnostic controversies, it should not be all that surprising that investigations of mechanisms of biofeedback therapy have led to muddled findings. It may even be premature to address therapy mechanisms until these pressing nosologic issues are resolved.

Finally, several biofeedback studies have found direction of physiologic control to be unimportant for treatment effectiveness (Andrasik & Holroyd, 1980; Cram, 1980; Gauthier, Bois, Allaire, & Drolet, 1981; Holroyd et al., 1984; Kewman & Roberts, 1983; Largen, Mathew, Dobbins, & Claghorn, 1981; Mullinix, Norton, Hack, & Fishman, 1978), raising questions about the specificity of biofeedback therapy. The absence of clear-cut relationships between biofeedback treatment indices and symptom change has led to speculations that cognitive and behavioral factors may underlie therapeutic effectiveness of biofeedback for a substantial proportion of patients (Holroyd & Penzien, 1983). Holroyd et al.'s (1984) study provides direct support for this conclusion. An alternative hypothesis for biofeedback, that conditioning of any type reduces lability in the target physiological response system and thus stabilizes physiology (Gauthier et al., 1981), is plausible but awaits empirical study.

Pediatric Headache

Prevalence studies reveal that a sizeable proportion of children are troubled by headaches. Headache has been found to occur in very young children, and by the age of 7, as many as 40% of all children may have experienced headache on a recurrent basis (once or more per month). Incidence of headache gradually but steadily increases throughout adolescence, as revealed in Figure 2 taken from Bille's (1962) extensive monograph. Recently completed longitudinal studies suggest, contrary to earlier speculations, that the majority of children with severe migraine may not outgrow their symptoms, but rather continue them into adulthood (Bille, 1981; Sillanpaa, 1983). Bille (1981) followed a sample of 73 children, all of whom had pronounced symptoms of migraine prior to the age of 6. Headache status was assessed on several occasions over a remarkable 23-year period (see Figure 3). At the last follow-up assessment, when all subjects had reached the minimum age of 30, 60% were still significantly troubled by migraine

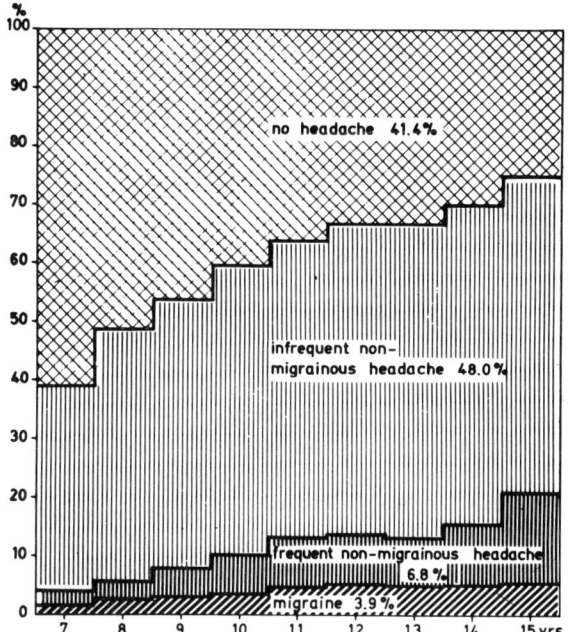

Figure 2. Occurrence and type of headache among 8,993 school children in Uppsala and percentage distribution between ages 7 and 15. Reproduced with permission from "Migraine in Childhood and Its Prognosis" by Bo Bille, 1981, *Cephalalgia, 1,*72.

headache. A significant effect emerged for gender in that headaches were retained by 70% of females but by 50% of males ($p < .05$). In either event, the long-term prognosis for pediatric migraine is rather bleak. Studies have yet to carefully map out the prevalence and course of pediatric tension headache.

Treatment studies for pediatric headache sufferers have lagged far behind those for adults. Diamond and Franklin's (1975) collection of uncontrolled case studies stood as the only biofeedback report for several years. More recently several additional reports have appeared and all reveal pronounced treatment effects (see Andrasik, Blake, & McCarran, 1986, for a review). Over the past few years we have been engaged in a large treatment trial comparing biofeedback and relaxation training, which also incorporates a treatment crossover component to investigate differential treatment responding. A no-treatment procedure was selected as the control condition to avoid certain ethical objections associated with pseudotherapy procedures. Both treatments incorporate elements of discrimination training (adapted from the work of Gainer, 1978), augmented home practice (portable biofeedback trainers or relaxation tapes), parental involvement, fading of treatment appointments over time, and a coping emphasis—all designed to facilitate initial treatment effects and promote mainte-

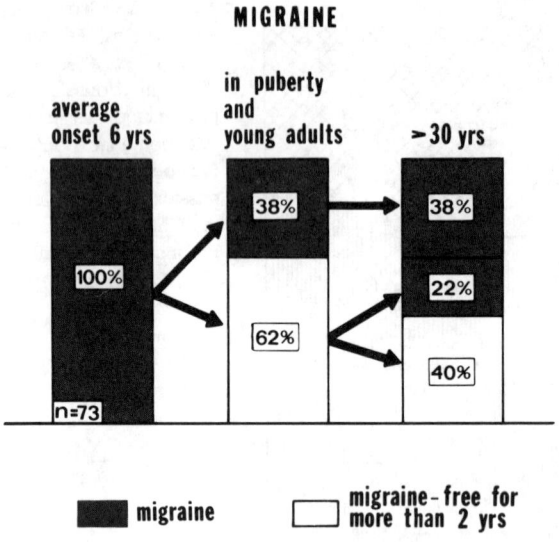

Figure 3. Seventy-three school children with "more pronounced" migraine followed-up during 23 years. Reproduced with permission from "Migraine in Childhood and Its Prognosis" by Bo Bille, 1981, Cephalalgia, 1, 74.

nance over time. The final analyses have yet to be completed, but interim evaluations reveal both treatments produce improvements well in excess of those found in the meta-analyses reported in Table 1 for adult patients and that the results are enduring for two years. The results were so favorable that few children have been available to enter the treatment crossover portion of the project. Children's increased enthusiasm, quicker rate of learning, enhanced confidence in "special abilities," fewer prior treatment failures, reduced chronicity, and reduced skepticism about self-control procedures are among the factors speculated to account for the increased treatment responsiveness found for them (Attanasio et al., 1985). Control subjects changed little during the waiting-list period. The only study to include a pseudotherapy control with children to date found those children with severe forms of migraine improved about only one-third as a result (Richter et al., 1986).

Alternative Therapy Delivery Modes

The number of individuals experiencing severe, recurrent headache (Leviton, 1978) vastly exceeds the capabilities of experienced therapists to treat them. This realization has led researchers to experiment with alternative, more time-efficient ways to deliver treatment without substantial loss in effectiveness. In early research conducted by the author (Andrasik & Holroyd, 1980; Holroyd, Andrasik, & Noble, 1980), biofeedback was administered in dyads for reasons of convenience. Outcomes obtained from these two studies appeared to be similar to those obtained when biofeedback was administered individually, but no direct comparisons were attempted back then. Recently, investigators have begun to study more time-efficient delivery modes in controlled fashion.

Alternate delivery models have been of two types—group administration or reduced laboratory contact. All but one investigation of effectiveness of group administration have involved multiple self-regulation therapies, which precludes evaluation of biofeedback by itself (Figueroa, 1982; Holroyd & Andrasik, 1978; Larsson & Melin, 1986; Williamson et al., 1984). The remaining study (Cote, Gauthier, & Cote, 1986) found equivalent rates of improvement for migraineurs administered thermal biofeedback either individually or in a small-group format (comprised of four to five patients).

In the second approach, time spent in the clinic or laboratory is markedly reduced with much of the learning taking place in the patient's home. Instructional aids (manuals and audiocassettes) are typically prepared to augment therapy. Implementing treatment largely out of a patient's home is believed to have a number of advantages, among them being reduced cost to patients (in terms of time, travel, and fees), greater availability for patients, and possible facilitation of maintenance effects (Glasgow & Rosen, 1978; Stokes & Bair, 1977). Most of the evaluations of reduced contact delivery models have similarly focused either on biofeedback combined with other forms of self-regulatory therapies or other forms of treatment in exclusion of biofeedback, the latter presumably occurring because of prohibitive equipment costs and technical complexities of biofeedback (Attanasio, Andrasik, & Blanchard, 1987; Blanchard et al., 1985a; Kohlenberg & Cahn, 1981; Tobin, Holroyd, Baker, & Reynolds, 1986).

Burke and Andrasik (1987) recently pilot-tested two ways to administer biofeedback from a reduced therapy contact model as a treatment for childhood migraine. In one condition parents served as therapists; in the other, children attempted to administer most of the treatment on their own. Both treatments were conducted under supervision of a therapist, but with markedly reduced contact (3 hours of therapist time vs. 10). Follow-up data collected through one year revealed similar effectiveness by both home-based treatment procedures; effectiveness rivaled that obtained by children treated in a standard, office-based procedure which was conducted for purposes of comparison. As technology advances and biofeedback units become cheaper, more portable, and easier to use (see Bischoff & Müller, this volume), research will no doubt become more active in this area.

References

Ad Hoc Committee on Classification of Headache (1962). Classification of headache. *Journal of the American Medical Association, 179,* 717—718.
Ad Hoc Committee of the International Headache Society (1987). *Proposed classification and diagnostic criteria for headache disorders, cranial neuralgias and facial pain.* Copenhagen: B. Stougaard Jensen.
Ahles, T.A., King, A., & Martin, J.E. (1984). EMG biofeedback during dynamic movement as a treatment for tension headache. *Headache, 24,* 41—44.
Ala-Hurula, V., Myllyla, V., & Hokkanen, E. (1982). Ergotamine abuse: Results of ergotamine discontinuation, with special reference to plasma concentration. *Cephalalgia, 2,* 189—195.
American Psychiatric Association (1980). *Biofeedback: Task force report number 19.* Washington, DC: American Psychiatric Association.
Andrasik, F., Blake, D.D., & McCarran, M.S. (1996). A biobehavioral analysis of pediatric headache. In N.A. Krasnegor, J.D. Arasteh, & M.F. Cataldo (Eds.), *Child health behavior: A behavioral pediatrics perspective* (pp. 394—434). New York: Wiley and Sons.
Andrasik, F., & Blanchard, E.B. (1987). The biofeedback treatment of tension headache. In J.P. Hatch, J.G. Fisher, & J.D. Rugh (Eds.), *Biofeedback: Studies in clinical efficacy* (pp. 281—321). New York: Plenum Press.
Andrasik, F., Blanchard, E.B., Arena, J.G., Saunders, N.L., & Barron, K.D. (1982). Psychophysiology of recurrent headache: Methodological issues and new empirical findings. *Behavior Therapy, 13,2* 407—429.
Andrasik, F., Blanchard, E.B., Neff, D.F., & Rodichok, L.D. (1984). Biofeedback and relaxation training for chronic headache: A controlled comparison of booster treatments and regular contacts for long-term maintenance. *Journal of Consulting and Clinical Psychology, 52,* 609—615.
Andrasik, F., & Holroyd, K.A. (1980). A test of specific and non-specific effects in the biofeedback treatment of tension headache. *Journal of Consulting and Clinical Psychology, 48,* 575—586.
Andrasik, F., & Holroyd, K.A. (1983). Specific and nonspecific effects in the biofeedback treatment of tension headache: 3-year follow-up. *Journal of Consulting and Clinical Psychology, 51,* 634—636.
AASH Board of Directors (1978). American Association for the Study of Headache: Biofeedback therapy. *Headache, 18,* 107.
Attanasio, V., Andrasik, F., & Blanchard, E.B. (1987). Cognitive therapy and relaxation training in muscle contraction headache: Efficacy and cost-effectiveness. *Headache, 27,* 254—260.
Attanasio, V., Andrasik, F., Burke, E.J., Blake, D.D., Kabela, E., & McCarran, M.S. (1985). Clinical issues in utilizing biofeedback with children. *Clinical Biofeedback and Health, 8,* 134—141.
Bakal, D.A., Kaganov, J.A., & Demjen, S. (1983). Headache assessment from a severity perspective. In K.A. Holroyd, B. Schlote & H. Zenz (Eds.), *Perspectives in research on headache* (pp. 45—55). Toronto, Lewiston, NY: C.J. Hogrefe.
Barlow, D.H., Hayes, S.C., & Nelson, R.O. (1984). *The scientist practitioner: Research and accountability in clinical and educational settings.* New York: Pergamon Press, 1984.
Bille, B. (1962). Migraine in school children. *Acta Paediatrica, 51* (supplement 136), 1—151.
Bille, B. (1981). Migraine in childhood and its prognosis. *Cephalalgia, 1,* 71—75.
Bischoff, C., & Traue, H.C. (1983). Myogenic headache. In K.A. Holroyd, B. Schlote & H. Zenz (Eds.), *Perspectives in research on headache* (pp. 66—90). Toronto/Lewiston, NY: C.J. Hogrefe.

Blanchard, E.B., & Andrasik, F. (1987). Biofeedback treatment of vascular headache. In J.P. Hatch, J.G. Fisher, & J.D. Rugh (Eds.), *Biofeedback: Studies in clinical efficacy* (pp. 1—79). New York: Plenum Press.

Blanchard, E.B., Andrasik, F., Ahles, T.A., Teders, S.J., & O'Keefe, D. (1980). Migraine and tension headache: A meta-analytic review. *Behavior Therapy, 11,* 613—631.

Blanchard, E.B., Andrasik, F., Appelbaum, K.A., Evans, D.D., Jurish, S.E., Teders, S.J., Rodichok, L.D., & Barron, K.D. (1985). The efficacy and cost-effectiveness of minimal-therapist-contact, non-drug treatments of chronic migraine and tension headache. *Headache, 25,* 214—220.

Blanchard, E.B., Andrasik, F., Evans, D.D., Neff, D.F., Appelbaum, K.A., & Rodichok, L.D. (1985). Behavioral treatment of 250 chronic headache patients: A clinical replication series. *Behavior Therapy, 16,* 308—327.

Blanchard, E.B., Andrasik, F., Jurish, S.E., & Teders, S.J. (1982). The treatment of cluster headache with relaxation and thermal biofeedback. *Biofeedback and Self-Regulation, 7,* 185—191.

Blanchard, E.B., Andrasik, F., Neff, D.F., Teders, S.J., Pallmeyer, T.P., Arena, J.G., Jurish, S.E., Saunders, N.L., Ahles, T.A., & Rodichok, L.D. (1982). Sequential comparisons of relaxation training and biofeedback in the treatment of three kinds of headche or, the machines may be necessary some of the time. *Behaviour Research and Therapy, 20,* 469—481.

Blanchard, E.B., Guarnieri, P., Andrasik, F., Neff, D.F., & Rodichok, L.D. (1987). Two-, three-, and four-year prospective follow-up on the behavioral treatment of chronic headache. *Journal of Consulting and Clinical Psychology, 55,* 257—259.

Blanchard, E.B., O'Keefe, D.M., Neff, D., Jurish, S., & Andrasik, F. (1981). Interdisciplinary agreement in the diagnosis of headache types. *Journal of Behavioral Assessment, 3,* 5—9.

Bruhn, P., Olesen, J., & Melgaard, B. (1979). Controlled trial of EMG feedback in muscle contraction headache. *Annals of Neurology, 6,* 34—36.

Budzynski, T., Stoyva, J., & Adler, C. (1970). Feedback-induced relaxation: Application to tension headache. *Journal of Behavior Therapy and Experimental Psychiatry, 1,* 205—211.

Budzynski, T.H., Stoyva, J.M., Adler, C.S., & Mullaney, D.J. (1973). EMG biofeedback and tension headache: A controlled outcome study. *Psychosomatic Medicine, 35,* 484—496.

Burke, E.J., & Andrasik, F. (1987). *Home- versus clinic-based treatments for pediatric migraine headache: Results of treatment through one-year follow-up.* Manuscript under review.

Cote, G., Gauthier, J., & Cote, A. (1986). *The treatment of migraine headache: A comparison of group versus individual biofeedback training.* Paper presented at the annual meeting of the Association for Advancement of Behavior Therapy, Chicago, Illinois, November.

Cram, J.R. (1980). EMG biofeedback and the treatment of tension headaches: A systematic analysis of treatment components. *Behavior Therapy, 11,* 699—710.

Diagnostic and Therapeutic Technology Asssessment (1983). Biofeedback. *Journal of the American Medical Association, 250,* 2381.

Diamond, S., & Franklin, M. (1975). Biofeedback: Choice of treatment in childhood migraine. In W. Luthe & F. Antonelli (Eds.), *Therapy in psychosomatic medicine, Vol. 4.* Rome: Autogenic Therapy.

Diamond, S., & Montrose, D. (1984). The value of biofeedback in the treatment of chronic headache: A four-year retrospective study. *Headache, 24,* 5—18.

Figueroa, J.L. (1982). Group treatment of chronic tension headaches. *Behavior Modification, 6,* 229—239.

Ford, M.R., Stroebel, C.F., Strong, P., & Szarek, B.L. (1983). Quieting response training: Long-term evaluation of a clinical biofeedback practice. *Biofeedback and Self-Regulation, 8,* 265—278.

Gainer, J.C. (1978). Temperature discrimination training in the biofeedback treatment of migraine headache. *Journal of Behavior Therapy and Experimental Psychiatry, 9*, 185—188.

Gauthier, J., Bois, R., Allaire, D., & Drolet, M. (1981). Evaluation of skin temperature biofeedback training at two different sites for migraine. *Journal of Behavioral Medicine, 4*, 407—419.

Gerhards, F., Rojahn, J., Boxan, K., Gnade, C., Petrik, M., & Florin, I. (1983). Biofeedback versus cognitive stress-coping therapy in migraine headache patients: A preliminary analysis of a comparative study. In K.A. Holroyd, B. Schlote & H. Zenz (Eds.), *Perspectives in research on headache* (pp. 163—170). Toronto/Lewiston, NY: C.J. Hogrefe.

Glasgow, R.E., & Rosen, G.M. (1978). Behavioral bibliotherapy: A review of self-help behavior therapy manuals. *Psychological Bulletin, 85*, 1—22.

Haber, J.D., Kuczmierczyk, A.R., & Adams, H.E. (1985). Tension headaches: Muscle overactivity or psychogenic pain. *Headache, 25*, 23—29.

Haynes, S.N. (1980). Muscle contraction headache: A psychophysiological perspective of etiology and treatment. In S.N. Haynes & L.R. Gannon (Eds.), *Psychosomatic disorders: A psychophysiological approach to etiology and treatment*. New York: Gardner.

Holroyd, K.A. (1986). Recurrent headache. In K. Holroyd & T. Creer (Eds.), *Self-management of chronic disease: Handbook of clinical interventions and research* (pp. 373—413). New York: Academic Press.

Holroyd, K.A., & Andrasik, F. (1978). Coping and the self-control of chronic tension headache. *Journal of Consulting and Clinical Psychology, 46*, 1036—1045.

Holroyd, K.A., & Andrasik, F. (1982). Do the effects of cognitive therapy endure? A two-year follow-up of tension headache sufferers treated with cognitive therapy or biofeedback. *Cognitive Therapy and Research, 6*, 325—333.

Holroyd, K.A., Andrasik, F., & Noble, J. (1980). A comparison of EMG biofeedback and a credible pseudotherapy in treating tension headache. *Journal of Behavioral Medicine, 3*, 29—39.

Holroyd, K.A., Andrasik, F., & Westbrook, T. (1977). Cognitive control of tension headache. *Cognitive Therapy and Research, 1*, 121—133.

Holroyd, K.A., & Penzien, D.B. (1983). EMG biofeedback and tension headache: Therapeutic mechanisms. In K.A. Holroyd, B. Schlote & H. Zenz (Eds.), *Perspectives in research on headache* (pp. 147—162). Toronto/Lewiston, NY: C.J. Hogrefe.

Holroyd, K.A., & Penzien, D.B. (1986). Client variables and the behavioral treatment of recurrent tension headache: A meta-analytic review. *Journal of Behavioral Medicine, 9*, 515—536.

Holroyd, K.A., Penzien, D.B., Hursey, K.G., Tobin, D.L., Rogers, L., Holm, J.E., Marcille, P.J., Hall, J.R., & Chila, A.G. (1984). Change mechanisms in EMG biofeedback training: Cognitive changes underlying improvements in tension headache. *Journal of Consulting and Clinical Psychology, 52*, 1039—1053.

Jacob, R.G., Turner, S.M., Szekely, B.C., & Eidelman, B.H. (1983). Predicting outcome of relaxation therapy in headaches: The role of "depression." *Behavior Therapy, 14*, 457—465.

Jay, G.W., Renelli, D., & Mead, T. (1984). The effects of propranolol and amitriptyline on vascular and EMG biofeedback training. *Headache, 24*, 56—69.

Kiesler, D.J. (1966). Some myths of psychotherapy research and the search for a paradigm. *Psychological Bulletin, 65*, 110—136.

Kewman, D., & Roberts, A.H. (1983). Skin temperature biofeedback and migraine headache: A double-blind study. *Biofeedback and Self-Regulation, 5*, 327—345.

Knapp, T.W. (1982). Treating migraine by training in temporal artery vasoconstriction and/or cognitive behavioral coping: A one-year follow-up. *Journal of Psychosomatic Research, 26*, 551—557.

Knapp, T.W., & Florin, I. (1981). The treatment of migraine headache by training in vasoconstriction of the temporal artery and a cognitive stress-coping training. *Behaviour Analysis and Modification, 4,* 267—274.
Kohlenberg, R.J., & Cahn, T. (1981). Self-help treatment for migraine headaches: A controlled outcome study. *Headache, 21,* 196—200.
Kudrow, L. (1982). Paradoxical effects of frequent analgesic use. In M. Critchley, A. Friedman, S. Gorini, & F. Sicuteri (Eds.), *Headache: Physiopathological and clinical concepts. Advances in Neurology, Vol. 33.* New York: Raven Press.
Largen, J.W., Mathew, R.J., Dobbins, K., & Claghorn, J.L. (1981). Specific and nonspecific effects of skin temperature control in migraine management. *Headache, 21,* 36—44.
Larsson, B., & Melin, L. (1986). Chronic headaches in adolescents: Treatment in a school setting with relaxation training as compared with information-contact and self-registration. *Pain, 25,* 325—336.
Leviton, A. (1978). Epidemiology of headache. In V.S. Schoenberg (Ed.), *Advances in neurology, Vol. 19* (pp. 341—352). New York: Raven Press.
Lynn, S.J., & Freedman, R.R. (1979). Transfer and evaluation of biofeedback treatment. In A. Goldstein & F. Kanfer (Eds.), *Maximizing treatment gains: Transfer enhancement in psychotherapy.* New York: Academic Press.
Martin, P.R. (1983). Behavioural research on headaches: Current status and future directions. In K.A. Holroyd, B. Schlote & H. Zenz (Eds.), *Perspectives in research on headache* (pp. 204—215). Toronto/Lewiston, NY: C.J. Hogrefe.
Mathew, N.T. (1981). Prophylaxis of migraine and mixed headache. A randomized controlled study. *Headache, 21,* 105—109.
Mathew, N.T., Reuveni, U., & Perez, F. (1987). Transformed or evolutive migraine. *Headache, 27,* 102—106.
Mullinix, V.J., Norton, B., Hack, S., & Fishman, M. (1978). Skin temperature biofeedback and migraine. *Headache, 17,* 242—244.
Paiva, T., Nunes, S., Moreira, A., Sontos, J., Teizeira, J., & Barbosa, A. (1982). Effects of frontalis EMG biofeedback and diazepam in the treatment of tension headache. *Headache, 22,* 216—220.
Philips, C. (1977). A psychological analysis of tension headache. In S. Rachman (Ed.), *Contributions to medical psychology, Vol. 1.* Oxford: Pergamon Press.
Rapoport, A., Sheftell, F., Baskin, S., & Weeks, R. (1984). *Analgesic rebound headache.* Paper presented at the meeting of the Migraine Trust, London, September.
Richter, I.L., McGrath, P.J., Humphreys, P.J., Goodman, J.T., Firestone, P., & Keene, D. (1986). Cognitive and relaxation treatment of pediatric migraine. *Pain, 25,* 195—203.
Saper, J.R. (1986). Changing perspectives on chronic headache. *Clinical Journal of Pain, 2,* 19—28.
Saper, J.R. (1987). Ergotamine dependency: A review. *Headache, 27,* 435-438.
Saper, J.R., & Jones, J.M. (1986). Ergotamine dependency. *Clinical Neuropharmacology, 9,* 244—256.
Sargent, J.D., Green, E.E., & Walters, E.D. (1972). The use of autogenic feedback training in a pilot study of migraine and tension headaches. *Headache, 12,* 120—124.
Sargent, J.D., Green, E.E., & Walters, E.D. (1973). Preliminary report on the use of autogenic feedback training in the treatment of migraine and tension headaches. *Psychosomatic Medicine, 35,* 129—135.
Schlote, B.M. (1983). Diagnostic procedures for the diagnosis of myogenic headache. In K.A. Holroyd, B. Schlote & H. Zenz (Eds.), *Perspectives in research on headache* (pp. 91—102). Toronto/Lewiston, NY: C.J. Hogrefe.

Sillanpaa, M. (1983). Changes in the prevalence of migraine and other headaches during the first seven school years. *Headache, 23,* 15—19.
Solbach, P., Sargent, J., & Coyne, L. (1984). Menstrual migraine headache: Results of a controlled, experimental, outcome study of nondrug treatments. *Headache, 24,* 75—78.
Sovak, N., Kunzel, M., Sternbach, R.A., & Dalessio, D.J. (1981). Mechanism of the biofeedback therapy of migraine: Volitional manipulation of the psychophysiological background. *Headache, 21,* 89—92.
Stokes, T.F., & Bair, D.M. (1977). An implicit technology of generalization. *Journal of Applied Behavior Analysis, 10,* 349—367.
Szekely, B., Botwin, D., Eidelman, B.H., Becker, M., Elman, N., & Schemm, R. (1986). Nonpharmacological treatment of menstrual headache: Relaxation biofeedback behavior therapy and person-centered insight therapy. *Headache, 26,* 86—92.
Tobin, D.L., Holroyd, K.A., Baker, A., & Reynolds, R. (1986). *Comparing minimal contact procedures for recurrent tension headache: Relaxation training vs. cognitive-behavior therapy.* Paper presented at the annual meeting of the Association for Advancement of Behavior Therapy, Chicago, Illinois, November.
Turkat, I.D., Brantley, P.J., Orton, K., & Adams, H.E. (1981). Reliability of headache diagnosis. *Journal of Behavioral Assessment, 3,* 1—4.
Weeks, R., Baskin, S., Rapoport, A., & Sheftell, F. (1984). *Reliability of headache diagnosis: A valid assumption or convenient fiction?* Paper presented at the 26th annual meeting of the American Association for the Study of Headache, San Francisco, CA, June.
Werder, D.S., Sargent, J.D., & Coyne, L. (1981). MMPI profiles of headache patients using self-regulation to control headache activity. *Headache, 21,* 164—169.
Williamson, D., Monguillot, J., Jarrell, P., Cohen, R., Pratt, M., & Blouin, D. (1984). Relaxation treatment of headache: Controlled evaluation of two group programs. *Behavior Modification, 8,* 407—424.
Wörz, R. (1983). Analgesic withdrawal in chronic pain treatment. In K.A. Holroyd, B. Schlote & H. Zenz (Eds.), *Perspectives in research on headache* (pp. 137—144). Toronto/Lewiston, NY: C.J. Hogrefe.

Portable EMG Biofeedback: A Single-Case Study with a Muscle Contraction Headache Sufferer

Claus Bischoff and Klaus-Jürgen Müller

EMG biofeedback is a very successful behavioral intervention in the treatment of tension headaches. The empirical results of Holroyd and colleagues would lead us to think that the therapeutical value of feedback is due to psychological learning (enhanced self-efficacy) rather than to physiological learning (modification of muscle activity). We argue that both mechanisms are influential. Physiological learning can only then take place (i) if it has an indication in the patient, i.e., if he/she suffers from true myogenic headache and shows deficits regarding the perception or control of muscular activity; and (ii) if the therapeutical setting allows for relevant physiological learning. Relevant physiological learning cannot take place in a relaxation chair but only at those moments of everyday life in which individuals should be sensitive to and control their muscle activity—in their individual stress- and emotion-provoking situations.

We describe a case study with a female patient who suffered from myogenic headache. The patient was treated with the help of a portable EMG biofeedback device during her working day. She was sensitized for static overload of the trapezius muscle and for the psychological meaning of the situations in which she statically overloaded this muscle. Tactile feedback was given when muscle tension continously exceeded an upper amplitude threshold longer than defined by a time threshold. Feedback stopped when the muscle activity remained under a lower amplitude threshold. The study had an ABAB design. Throughout the experimental phases the patient kept a diary on headaches, feelings of tension, and stress. Symptoms markedly declined during treatment. The level of muscular activity remained almost equally high; muscular dynamics increased. Consequences of the study for further research are discussed.

The two most detailed meta-analytical studies in the last years on behavioral medical interventions in tension headaches (Blanchard et al., 1980; Holroyd & Penzien, 1985) arrive at the clear consensus that EMG biofeedback is equivalent to, if not superior to, other methods of treatment. Contingent biofeedback, in which the feedback signal is a function of the patient's present muscle tension, has also definitely a greater effect as methods of pseudo-treatment, such as the keeping of a headache diary and noncontingent feedback. It still remains unexplained, however, what mechanisms are mainly responsible for the effective-

---

The research was carried out with the support of the German Research Foundation (DFG) in the Special Research Unit 129 ("Psychotherapeutic Processes") at the University of Ulm, FRG. The authors wish to thank F. Andrasik, J. Cram, E. Dahlinger, H.-J. Grünzig, P. Marschall, and H.C. Traue for their critical and constructive comments made on an earlier draft of this paper, and P. Zintl for the translation of the manuscript.

ness of biofeedback. Several studies showed that even patients who had learned about increasing muscle tension or the realization of a constant muscle tension through contingent biofeedback—and thus being of the opinion that they would relax—gained from the treatment (Andrasik & Holroyd, 1980, 1983; Holroyd et al., 1984). These results are contrary to the idea that the EMG biofeedback develops its effects on the basis of a physiological learning process, i.e., on the basis of a trained reduction of muscle tension. Furthermore, Holroyd and colleagues were repeatedly able to demonstrate empirically that patients who believe that they have successfully solved the biofeedback task profit much more from feedback training than patients who are accredited little success. The difference occurred independently of the actual work in training. "This raises the possibility that biofeedback training is effective largely because it provides subjects with contingent success experiences on a highly credible therapeutic task, not because it enables subjects to reduce EMG-levels" (Holroyd & Penzien, 1985, p. 25).

Yet it should be taken into consideration that it depends upon the conception of the study, its design, and its choice of patients as to what emphasis is placed on physiological learning. The studies mentioned maximize the possible influence of psychological factors, especially that of self-efficacy.

Biofeedback is beneficial in virtue of physiological learning only
(i) if physiological learning has an indication in the patient, and
(ii) if the therapeutical setting offers enough scope for relevant physiological learning.

ad (i): The question of indication has two components: First, do the patients examined really suffer from myogenic headaches, i.e., headaches that are caused by dysfunctionally working muscles? And does the biofeedback apply to the musculature causing the headaches? If this is not the case, then, for physiological reasons, it is nonsensical to hope for a relief of the symptoms by the reduction of muscle tension.

Previous tests on the mechanisms have not taken into account the myogeny of tension headaches. It cannot be ruled out that, for a number of patients, the headaches can be explained better with the operant conditioning model of pain (Fordyce, 1976) or as a depression equivalent. If there is no dysfunctional muscle activity, but rather a limitation of self-efficacy (as, for example, is often the case with depressive people), it is not surprising that the increase in self-efficacy through biofeedback is therapeutically more effective than the influence of the muscle activity.

The question of myogeny also affects the area of registration, that is, the musculature to which the feedback should be applied. In the standard version of biofeedback, the lead position is the forehead. Are the forehead, temples, and jaw muscles, which have been included in this registration (Basmajian, 1976), at all relevant to the patient's headache? Not necessarily with every patient. Whoever intends to bring about a physiological learning process in order to reduce the myogenic headache must train that muscle or those muscles whose activity directly affects the headache as, there are numerous indications that the relaxation of a muscle induced by biofeedback does not necessarily spread to untrained muscles (Friedlund et al., 1980, 1982). How then can the area of registration be sensibly established? Several possibilities are conceivable. Suggestions were the area with the strongest tension—in which case the question arises: Which "tension norm" one can refer to: the area of the strongest pains (Belar, 1979) and the area of registration preferred by the patient (Hudzinski, 1983). In our opinion the therapist should try to identify the probable focus of tension by taking the pattern of referred pains into consideration (Travell & Simons, 1983), and to apply biofeedback to the affected muscle.

Second, must the patients really learn what they ought to learn physiologically with biofeedback: increasing the perception of muscular tension and improving the ability to voluntarily control muscle tension? Not every myogenic headache sufferer has apriori a deficit in the ability of perception and control. One may be competent but not performant: one does not exploit one's own capabilities.

It is highly probable that, in comparison to other people, persons with myogenic headaches do not perceive their muscle tension quite as well. In group comparisons their sensitivity is reduced, and they are more cautious when evaluating their muscle tension (see Bischoff & Sauermann, in this volume). Empirical data on awareness do not exist. Interestingly enough, there is no evidence up to now that the ability to control muscle tension in persons suffering from myogenic headache is less developped than that in controls (Bischoff, 1989). These findings are based on groups' average means. Strictly speaking, with each patient in whom biofeedback is taken into consideration as a method of treatment for physiological reasons, it must be clarified in the individual behavior analysis whether his or her perceptual and control abilities need to be improved.

ad (ii): The possibility for relevant physiological learning: In our view, the perception of muscle tension is a crucial factor in the etiology of myogenic headache. Most of the time, as in walking, the CNS processes proprioceptive stimulation automatically. The stimuli do not become conscious. The awareness of proprioceptive stimuli is restricted above all to emotional states and states of physical and cognitive effort. In emotional states, patterns of proprioceptive stimuli act as an aid in decoding the quality of emotion called up (Gellhorn, 1964; Izard, 1977; Tomkins, 1980; LeDoux, 1984; Laird, 1984). In states of physical and cognitive effort, proprioceptive stimuli together with other interoceptively noticable bodily stimuli are stop signals, when the energetic resources of the body are dangerously close to becoming exhausted (Edwards et al., 1972; Mihevic, 1981). Therefore, the awareness of proprioceptive stimuli has an important function in the regulation of actions—of actions that take into account the needs and capacities of the body. Myogenic headache sufferers exhibit behavioral dysfunctions in both cases: They show an inhibition of emotional expression (Traue et al., 1985a; Traue, in this volume), and they tend to engage excessively in activities statically overloading the muscles of the neck and head area, as in typewriting or working in front of a screen (Robinson, 1980). In both cases, it is a matter of static overloading of the muscles which, according to studies dealing with physiology at work (Ulmer, 1985), with 15—20% of maximum contraction can already lead to pains. Most probably, the individual learns inhibition and overloading by operant conditioning (Bischoff & Traue, 1983). In both cases awareness of muscle tension loses its function. It is rather impairing, and is extinguished by operant conditioning, too. We think this is the reason for the perceptual deficit in myogenic headache sufferers.

Following these considerations it should be clear that the traditional EMG biofeedback procedure with the headache patient lying in the relaxation chair of the psychologist's consultation room is an incomplete therapeutic method. On the one hand, it is doubtful whether, in order to control headaches, these patients really have to learn to perceive such slight differences in tension which occur in the relaxation chair. More important is that they can distinguish between the increased muscle tension arising as a result of mental and physical work and emotionally charged situations from the state of relaxation. Biofeedback should help to achieve this. Seen from this point of view, feedback training in which patients tense their muscles and still believes they are relaxing them, as is realized as a control condition by the Holroyd group, on no account offers an opportunity for relevant physiological learning. On the other hand, traditional biofeedback does not sensitize the patients for the most "dangerous" type of muscle tension: for static overload. Moreover, a patient who is able to perceive muscle tension correctly when he or she focuses attention on it by instruction is not necessarily aware of muscle activity in everyday life. Finally, the patient is not confronted with the specific connections between muscle tension and the behaviors producing it—inhibition of emotional expression and excessive achievement behavior with respect to activities statically overloading the muscles of the neck and head region.

The limited possibilities of bringing about relevant physiological learning processes in patients through traditional biofeedback constitute a problem that, seen in another perspective, can also be interpreted as a problem of the transfer of training: Being able to improve the awareness and control of muscle tension through biofeedback in the relaxation chair does not mean that these abilities are readily present in critical everyday situations. The problem of the transfer of training is not new in EMG biofeedback. Various dimensions of transfer have been considered and examined. Patients have been instructed to do the biofeedback exercises not only at the therapist's but also at home (Kotses & Weiner, 1982; Reinking & Hutchings, 1981; Andrasik et al., 1984; Sargent, Solbach & Coyne, 1980; Libo & Arnold, 1983). They were instructed to achieve not only a low but also a constant muscle tension (Cram, 1980). Biofeedback was applied while the patient sat, stood, or walked around, or while imagining difficult situations or talking to the therapist (Ahles, King & Martin, 1984; Carrobles, Cardona & Santacreu, 1981). Hudzinski (1984) added a special "discrimination training" for the facial muscles. Four out of the five stated studies on home practice proved that this additional practice stabilized or even improved the success of the therapy. The regularity of the exercises at home does not, however, seem to be so important. The results concerning the other transfer dimensions generally show a tendency toward the superiority of biofeedback therapy that is not restricted to the traditional technique. On the other hand, the results are not sufficiently clear as to allow a final evaluation.

We have gone one step further and developped a portable device that gives the patient a biofeedback of muscle tension in everyday life. In order to gain experience with this method, we examined its effectiveness in a single-case study.

Method

Apparatus

The device consists of two small boxes: EMG module, the smaller box, and a processor and store unit (Figure 1). The modul amplifies the EMG signal, filters it with high- and low-pass filters (lower frequency limit 80 Hz, upper frequency limit 1000 Hz), and rectifies and integrates the signal. The programmable processor and store unit stores the EMG integrals and controls the delivery of the biofeedback signal. The patient wears the boxes on the belt or in the inside pocket of his/her jacket.

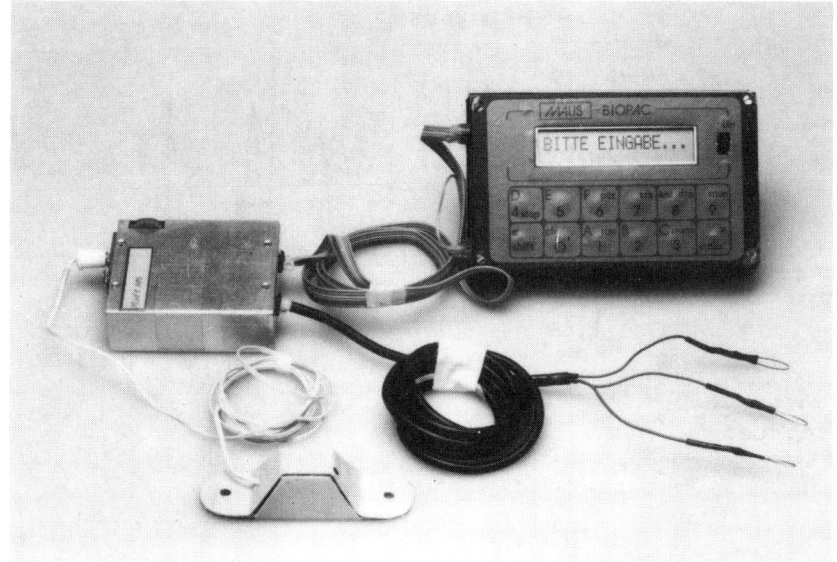

Figure 1. Portable EMG biofeedback device (Maus, Ludwigshafen, FRG).

During everyday life the patient should perceive the biofeedback signal, though the people one interacts with should *not* notice anything. This is attained by an electrical stimulator (see Figure 1, left front). The maximum stimulus intensity is 20 V with a current intensity of 200 µA. The stimulator delivers impulses modeling the level of muscle activity in two ways. Their frequency varies between 200 and 600 Hz, and they simultaneously are bundled up into impulse packages whose frequencies amount to 1/32 of the basic frequencies of the feedback stimulus. The patient receives the electrical stimulation at the back of the left arm via leads. At this place no efferent nerves are directly stimulated. The intensity of the stimulus is adjusted so that the patient clearly perceives it but does not find it to be unpleasant.

The delivery of the biofeedback signal is controlled by three thresholds that are programmable with the internal processor unit (cf. Figure 2). Feedback is released when the EMG integral continuously exceeds the upper amplitude threshold longer than defined by the time threshold. Feedback stops when the EMG integral remains under the lower amplitude threshold. The example in Figure 2 shows the delivery of feedback when the integral continously exceeds 50 µV/s longer than 4 minutes and the switching-off of the signal when the EMG drops below 20 µV/s.

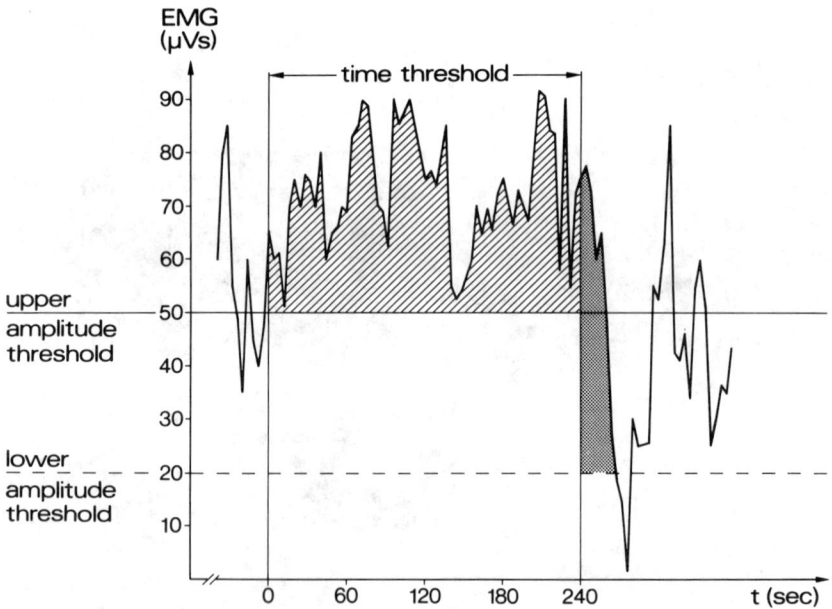

Figure 2. Interaction of time and amplitude thresholds of the portable EMG biofeedback device.

The upper amplitude threshold and the time threshold interact in such a way that biofeedback is delivered as soon as the muscle in question is about to become statically overloaded.

Subject

The patient is female, 33 years old, single; she works in an open-plan office of a health insurance company. She was selected as subject because it was known from a former psychophysiological field study (see Schlote, in this volume) that her subjective symptomatology clearly pointed to myogenic headache. In addition, she exhibited an extremely high trapezius muscle activity all day long, and muscle tension correlated significantly with headache intensity.

Behavior Analysis

Headache interview and headache questionnaire yield the following results: The patient suffers both from myogenic headaches and from migraines. Myogenic headache—bilateral feelings of tightness and pressure rising from the neck—occurs on working days almost daily. It starts early in the morning with low intensity, has a peak level at high noon, and becomes less intensive during the afternoon hours and in the evening. Besides changes in the weather, it is intensive work in front of a monitor screen, writing by hand, and typing which triggers the headaches. She often accumulates certain tasks of the same type, for instance filing, in order to attend to this matter at one go. On the other hand, headaches occur when she feels angry with a client but does not want to show her anger. Moreover, headaches are triggered by tense posture when driving a car. She thinks she is a very anxious motorist. The classical migraine attacks she suffers from in addition to this are limited to weekends and to menstruation. She only occasionally takes medication.

Headache History

Headache occurred for the first time with menarche. The symptoms intensified from the 17th year on, arrived at a maximum in the middle of her twenties, and have been decreasing for two years now. Two years ago both her mother and her sister-in-law died. This sounds paradoxical, but it is not. She lived in her parents' house until her mother's death. Her mother took over all duties for her at home, so she had a lot of time left to rack her brain why she couldn't find the right man to marry and settle down with. Years ago she had entered into two or three short love affairs which did not last because of her parents and her own high demands. In addition, she lacked and still lacks self-confidence in becoming acquainted with the opposite sex. Since her mother's death she has been living in her own apartment quite near her brother. In the morning and the evening hours she acts as a substitute mother and looks after both the children of her deceased sister-in-law.

Design

We used an ABAB-design for this single-case study (cf. Table 1) consisting of baseline phase 1 followed by treatment phase 1, baseline phase 2, and finally by treatment phase 2.

Table 1. Design of the single case study on portable EMG biofeedback.

	Baseline 1 (29 days)	Treatment 1 (13 days)	Baseline 2 (24 days)	Treatment 2 (11 days)
Headache Interview (MANOK & ZENZ)	X			
Headache Questionnaire (SCHLOTE)	X			
Diary (headache, feelings of tension and stress)	X ——————————————————————————— X			
Field registration of trapezius EMG	XXXXXX	XXXXXXXX	XXXXXX	XXXXXXXX
Field EMG-biofeedback of trapezius activity		XXXXXXXX		XXXXXXXX
Credibility scale (HOLROYD)				X

At the beginning of the first baseline phase I the first author interviewed the patient using the semistructured headache interview by Manok and Zenz (this volume), and the patient filled in the headache questionnaire by Schlote. The diagnostic information described above stems from these two diagnostic instruments. From the beginning to the end of the study the patient kept a diary on headaches, feelings of tension, and stress. Every other hour she rated these variables on a 10-point rating scale. A watch with hour signal reminded her to write down the recordings. On the back of the diary index card the patient registered medication intake and, during treatment phases, the forms of behavior eliciting biofeedback. The EMG of the upper trapezius muscle was measured in her office from 8 a.m. till 2 p.m. on six days during baselines and on eight days during treatment phases. During treatment phases EMG biofeedback was administered simultaneously to EMG registration. EMG registration and biofeedback referred to the upper trapezius muscle because the pattern of pain locations indicated that in this patient it was the activity of this muscle which was mostly responsible for the development of headaches (compare the data of the behavior analysis and the correspondent pain pattern described by Travell & Simons, 1984). The EMG of the right trapezius muscle was registered by surface leads with the bipolar standard lead position between the acromion and vertebra C7 (Zipp, 1982). The EMG was registered on the right side to avoid interference with the heart rate. The electrical stimulus was applied contralaterally to avoid undesired effects on the EMG registration.

Hypotheses

If the treatment is effective, headache activity should be most intensive in baseline 1, less intensive in baseline 2, even less intensive in treatment phase 1, and least intensive in treatment phase 2. The same should be true with respect to feelings of muscle tension and stress, and to EMG average level. Since the biofeedback treatment intends to reduce static muscular activity, it can be expected that the dynamics of muscle activity increase in reverse order of rank. Dynamic muscle activity most should markedly occur during treatment phases. Applying the nonparametric randomization test by Levin et al. (1978), the likelihood of the hypothesized orders of ranks is less than $p = .05$.

Treatment

At the beginning of a treatment day the patient was trained to control trapezius muscle activity with respect to the amplitude threshold valid for the respective day and a time threshold of one second. She tested postures and movements leading to biofeedback and those turning it off. As an aid for relaxation she used prolonged respiratory exhalation (Cappo & Holmes, 1984). (Strictly speaking, these instructions accentuate feedforward rather than feedback learning processes (LaCroix, 1981; Dunn et al., 1986). The patient selects and tries out responses already available to her and uses the vibratory information to confirm the assumption that these forms of behavior have the effect to reduce muscle tension.) Following these exercises, thresholds were adjusted so that the patient presumably would not receive more than 20 biofeedbacks during the 6 treatment hours. The time threshold was constantly 4 minutes.

Figure 3 shows a typical treatment day. As expected, headache intensity and the intensity of tension and stress feelings develop from small intensities in the early morning up to higher intensities in the course of the day, to decline in the evening hours. The peak values of the average EMG level per hour approximately parallel those of the subjective variables. The arrows pointing to the abscissa indicate the times biofeedback was delivered.

At the end of each treatment day, the therapist discussed the biofeedback events with the patient to find alternative behaviors that probably would not produce biofeedback. From the second treatment day on the patient got the impres-

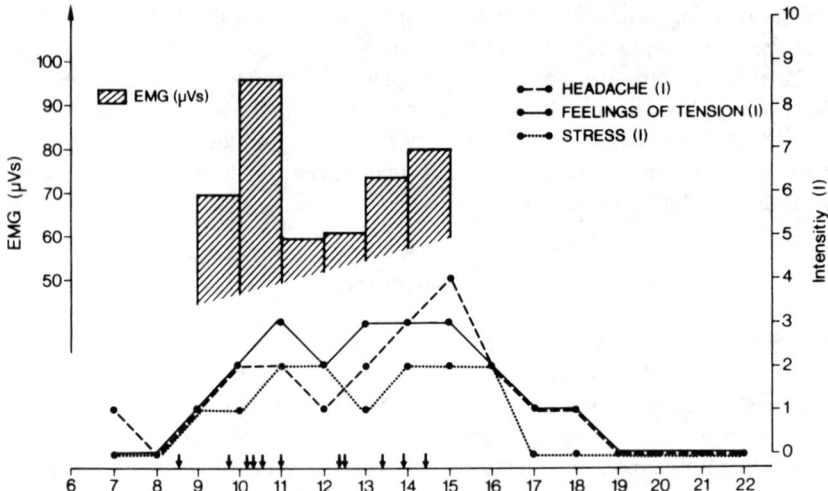

Figure 3. EMG, headache, and feelings of tension and stress during a typical day with field biofeedback.

sion of being able to predict correctly biofeedback events; from the fourth day on she tried to avoid biofeedback by behaving at the right time in the way discussed before.

Table 2 sums up the behaviors that elicited biofeedback during both treatment periods. The bulk of biofeedback events belongs to the category of writing activities. Another interesting category is conversations with colleagues and clients. Characteristic of conversations leading to feedback were arising feelings of anger and their immediate inhibition.

Results

Headache Activity

We computed three indices of headache activity: the headache density p.d., the number of hours with headache p.d., and the maximum headache intensity p.d. The daily density is the sum of the 16 intensity ratings of that day. The patient had five migraine attacks in the course of the study. They were excluded from data analysis. There is a marked improvement in the headaches from baseline 1 to treatment 1 (cf. Table 3). As hypothesized, there is a tendency of increasing symptoms in baseline 2; but in contrast to our prediction, the second treatment phase does result in a further alleviation of the symptoms.

For tension and stress feelings, we computed densities, too. The results are quite similar: marked reduction from baseline 1 to treatment 1—a reduction continuing in baseline 2—and stagnation in treatment phase 2 (Table 3).

Table 2. Behaviors eliciting EMG-biofeedback (records of the patient)

Behaviors eliciting biofeedback	Frequency
Writing	
– by hand (desk)	21
– by hand (conference record)	8
– type	30
– screen	8
– calculator	1
Reading	1
Filing	8
Unwrapping	1
Conversations with	
– collegues	11
– clients (counter, telephone)	9
Lunch break (eating, shopping)	16
Unfavorable postures	4
?	28

Table 3. Diary indices and EMG-parameters during baseline and treatment phases

	Baseline 1	Treatment 1	Baseline 2	Treatment 2
Headache density p. d. (Σ intensity ratings p. d.)	17.1	7.8	9.6	9.3
Number of hours with headache p. d.	10.4	5.2	5.9	6.3
Maximum headache intensity p. d.	2.7	1.9	1.4	2.0
Density of tension feelings p. d. (Σ intensity ratings p. d.)	24.7	15.2	11.0	9.7
Density of stress ratings p. d. (Σ intensity ratings p. d.)	11.5	8.9	3.8	4.3
EMG-parameters (μVs): Average/hours	87.6	92.6	96.1	101.7
Mean square of successive differences/hours	894.9	1206.4	1536.4	1705.1

Muscle Activity

The average hourly EMG level of the patient is very high from the beginning—even when compared with the EMG level of other myogenic headache sufferers in the same situation (cf. Schlote, in this volume), and it remains high throughout all the experimental periods. There is even a trend toward an increase. This result clearly contradicts the hypothesis. On the other hand and in line with our expectations, a progressing dynamization of muscle activity takes place from one phase to the following. As index of static vs. dynamic muscle activity, the successive differences of the 4-second EMG integrals were computed, squared and averaged.

Discussion

We start with the EMG results: Biofeedback does not lower the general level of muscle activity. Nevertheless, levels of muscle activity are correlated with headache. The correlation between the hourly headache intensity ratings and the averaged EMG integrals of the hour immediately before the rating is $r = .54$. This finding replicates the result of the previous study with the same patient. This may indicate that the average means of whole periods are measures that are not sensitive enough to grasp the relevant aspects of single headache episodes. In any case, the effectiveness of our biofeedback training cannot be explained by the so-called cultivated low arousal which Stoyva and Budzynski (1974) considered to be the cause of feedback-induced pain reduction.

The dynamization is not surprising—it was explicitly trained by means of biofeedback. Because of the simultaneously increasing EMG level, one could argue that dynamization is an artifact. Actually, hourly EMG levels and corresponding successive differences correlate positively with $r = .57$. But analysis of covariance with the EMG levels as covariate nonetheless confirms the hypothesis of progressing dynamization $(F = 19.01 > F(3,156; 99\%) = 3.9)$. Therefore, dynamization appears to be a process in its own right.

Why does the second treatment phase not lead to an additional pain reduction? The headache problem possibly has aspects that are not controllable by feedback treatment. Perhaps the patient has already learned all the skills in the first treatment phase which can be learned by the biofeedback training, and which are effective in avoiding headaches; the second training cannot further improve these skills. Indeed, several investigators (see Yates, 1980) have pointed out that learning by biofeedback differs from other learning processes regarding the characteristics of acquisition and extinction. The individual learns biofeedback-induced control of body processes very quickly and completely and often maintains the control ability without further practice. Therefore, it is not surprising that repeating classical biofeedback for more than about 12 sessions does not lead to an increased benefit of training (Chapman, 1986). With respect to time consumption, 12 sessions of classical biofeedback correspond to about two treatment days with field biofeedback. Inasmuch as the observations regarding the learning processes in classical biofeedback are valid for field biofeedback as well, an ABAB design even proves to be unsuitable for testing the effectiveness of the new method. A second explanation: Conditions are not constant in a therapy lasting a quarter of a year. At the end of baseline 2, the patient fell in love. She had had no experience in love affairs for some 15 years and became a bit disturbed by her feelings. In addition, the affair turned out to be complicated for several reasons. Therefore, it may not be surprising that the tiny electrical feedback impulses were helpless against Cupid's arrows.

The positive effects of biofeedback on psychological variables has frequently been described in the literature referring to headaches (Andrasik et al., 1984; Bell et al., 1983; Blanchard et al., 1986; Cox & Thomas 1981; Cox, Lefebvre & Hobbs, 1982; Gerber et al., 1983). Indications of such changes were also present in the course of the biofeedback therapy with the patient in our study. In the *Biographical Inventory of Behavioral Disturbances* (Jäger et al., 1976), a reduction of neuroticism becomes apparent (from stanine 6 to 4). The patient also finds her social situation not such a strain as before therapy (reduction of the stanine score from 6 to 4). With headache patients the locus of control as well as the health locus of control is often external. Psychological therapy, therefore, often results in, or aims at, increasing self-responsiblity, i.e., a changing of control attributions toward internal control (Funke, 1988). In contrast to this, at the beginning of therapy our patient had an extremely internal locus of control (stanine 7 in the *IPC Questionnaire* by Krampen, 1981). This corresponded with her rejecting the possibility that she could be influenced by other powerful people (stanine 1) or by factors of chance (stanine 2). This self-concept—reminding one of the greek mythological figure antaeus—became "normal" in the course of the therapy (stanine 5 for the scale "internal control," stanine 2 for the scale "powerful others," and stanine 4 for the scale "chance." The result was therefore a more modest attitude in the evalution of ones own possible influences—which not only reflects a more realistic self-concept, but may also be relieving and convey composure.

All things considered, the results are encouraging. The patient's complaints—headaches and feelings of tension—decreased markedly during treatment. The same is true for her feelings of stress. The patient's ratings on Holroyd's credibility scale showed that she is convinced that the treatment will help her to reduce future headaches (score 3 on the 5-point Likert scale). The treatment effect was so convincing for her that she would in any case recommend the training to friends who suffer from headache, and she thinks that it is very important to make the treatment available to other patients experiencing tension headaches. However, it is worth considering that according to empirical findings, certain characteristics of the patient as well as of the therapeutic arrangements would favor a success in the treatment right from the start: the patient is young and female (Holroyd & Penzien, 1985), there are no signs of depression

(Blanchard et al., 1985; Cox, Lefebvre & Hobbs, 1982; Jacob et al., 1983), the headaches vary in intensity and are restricted to situations (Bakal et al., 1981; Blanchard et al., 1982; Jacob et al., 1983). Apart from that, it was the experimenter who offered the training to the patient and the "experimental group" was as small as possible (Holroyd & Penzien, 1985).

The assessment of the causal factors is even more difficult in field biofeedback than in traditional feedback, simply because the number of possible causal factors is greater. The device itself already gives three types of feedback. In starting the biofeedback signal, it points to the fact that now the muscle is statically contracted. By means of the prickly sensation, which proportionally depicts muscle tension, it reports back the muscle activity of the moment, and through the switching off of the feedback stimulus it shows that the readings are below a critical threshold of relaxation. The psychophysiological meaning of the feedback process is even more complex. The triggering off of the feedback signal indicates that a certain motoric behavior, of the operant or reflex type, is connected to static contractions. The feedback signal itself reveals the degrees of tension the present behavior is producing. The switching off of the signal indicates that a certain behavior has lead to relaxation. Different learning objectives are combined with these feedback components. Through the triggering off of the signal the patient can learn an awareness of static muscle activities. The feedback signal varying with the muscle tension enables him to sharpen his sensitivity toward muscle tension. If the feedback signal no longer appears, it teaches the patient which of the endeavours has been successful in regulating muscle activities in the direction of relaxation. Field biofeedback therefore places the feedback task in a behavioral context, aiming at physiological learning by means of psychology. This therapeutic rationale to give up the idea that field biofeedback is a method of relaxation. It is not the patient's task to make the feedback signal disappear as soon as possible through directed relaxation, but rather to be aware of the behavior that helps him or her to overcome, better than before, the strain that has led to the triggering off of the signal in the first place. In some cases the best possibility of coping consists of relaxation or physiotherapy exercises. In other situations it would be better *not* to suppress the feelings that have arisen in the situation, but to express oneself freely and confidently. Patients are possibly not confident in this situation, so that it is advisable, through an appropriate behavioral training, to improve their assertiveness. After static overload of the muscles those behaviors are adequate that guarantee the regeneration of the organism. The psychotherapeutic task consists of finding out, together with the patients, just what prevented them up to now from allowing themselves to regenerate.

Biofeedback is not a scientific invention. Internal feedback loops are the way the organism regulates himself. Physiological and biochemical processes can be excellently described with cybernetic models. Most of the self-regulating processes occur unconsciously; consciousness appears to be responsible for the malfunctions. Interoceptive detection of bodily processes in emotions and states of physical or intellectual stress act as internal feedback signals that stimulate behaviors compensating the existing imbalances. Also, pain as well as general feelings of uneasiness are normally feedback signals that show the individual that there is a dysfunction that must be eliminated. These signals often arise when the weaker interocepts associated with emotions and stress have been ignored for a period of time. It is these peculiarities of self-regulation that caused Schwartz (1977) to describe the organism as a "health care system." Seen in this light, external biofeedback with a device is only then of value in the treatment of headaches or, generally speaking, of psychophysiological disorders if it supports the self-regulation of the organisms. Its contribution must be to install the internal feedback signals in their original function.

References

Ahles, T.A., King, A., & Martin, J.E. (1984). EMG biofeedback during dynamic movement as a treatment for tension headache. *Headache, 24,* 41—44.

Andrasik, F., Blanchard, E.B., Neff, D.F., & Rodichok, L.D. (1984). Biofeedback and relaxation training for chronic headache: A controlled comparison of booster treatment and regular contacts for long-term maintenance. *Journal of Consulting and Clinical Psychology, 52,* 609—615.

Andrasik, F., & Holroyd, K.A. (1980). A test of specific and nonspecific effects in the biofeedback treatment of tension headache. *Journal of Consulting and Clinical Psychology, 48,* 575—586.

Andrasik, F., & Holroyd, K.A. (1983). Specific and nonspecific effects in the biofeedback treatment of tension headache: 3-year follow-up. *Journal of Consulting and Clinical Psychology, 51,* 634—636.

Bakal, D.A., Demjen, S., & Kaganov, F.A. (1981). Cognitive behavioral treatment of chronic headache. *Headache, 21,* 81—86.

Basmajian, J.V. (1976). Facts versus myths in EMG biofeedback. *Biofeedback and Self-Regulation, 1,* 369—371.

Belar, C.D. (1979). A comment on Silver and Blanchard's (1978) review of the treatment of tension headaches by EMG feedback and relaxation training. *Journal of Behavioral Medicine, 2,* 215—220.

Bell, N.W., Abramowitz, S.I., Folkins, C.H., Spensley, J., & Hutchinson, G.L. (1983). Biofeedback, brief psychotherapy and tension headache. *Headache, 23,* 162—173.

Bischoff, C. (1989). *Wahrnehmung der Muskelspannung.* Göttingen: Hogrefe.

Bischoff, C., & Traue, H.C. (1983). Myogenic headache. In K.A. Holroyd, B. Schlote, & H. Zenz (Eds.), *Perspectives in research on headache* (pp. 66—90). Toronto/Lewiston, NY: C.J. Hogrefe.

Blanchard, E.B., Andrasik, F., Ahles, T.A., Teders, S.J., & O'Keefe, D. (1980). Migraine and tension headache: A meta-analytic review. *Behavior Therapy, 11,* 613—631.

Blanchard, E.B., Andrasik, F., Appelbaum, K.A., Evans, D.D., Meyers, P., & Barron, K.D. (1986). Three studies of the psychological changes in chronic headache patients associated with biofeedback and relaxation therapies. *Psychosomatic Medicine, 48,* 73—83.

Blanchard, E.B., Andrasik, F., Evans, D.D., Appelbaum, K.A., & Rodichok, L.D. (1985). Be-

havioral treatment of 250 chronic headache patients: A clinical replication series. *Behavior Therapy, 16,* 308—327.
Blanchard, E.B., Andrasik, F., Neff, D.F., Teders, S.J., Pallmeyer, T.P., Arena, J.G., Jurish, S.E., Saunders, N.L., Ahles, T.A., & Rodichok, L.D. (1982). Sequential comparisons of relaxation training and biofeedback in the treatment of three kinds of chronic headache or, the machines may be necessary some of the time. *Behavior Research and Therapy, 20,* 469—481.
Cappo, B.M., & Holmes, D.S. (1984). The utility of prolonged respiratory exhalation for reducing physiological arousal in non-threatening and threatening situations. *Journal of Psychosomatic Research, 28,* 265—273.
Carrobles, J.A., Cardona, A., & Santacreu, J. (1981). Shaping and generalization procedures in the EMG-biofeedback treatment of tension headaches. *British Journal of Clinical Psychology, 20,* 49—56.
Chapman, S.L. (1986). A review and clinical perspective on the use of EMG and thermal biofeedback for chronic headaches. *Pain, 27,* 1—43.
Cox, D.J., Lefebvre, R.C., & Hobbs, W.R. (1982). Ancillary symptoms in the biofeedback treatment of headaches. *Headache, 22,* 213—215.
Cox, D., & Thomas, D. (1981). Relationship between headaches and depression. *Headache, 21,* 261—263.
Cram, J.R. (1980). EMG biofeedback and the treatment of tension headaches: A systematic analysis of treatment components. *Behavior Therapy, 11,* 699—710.
Dunn, T.G., Gillig, S.E., Ponsor, S.E., & Weil, N. (1986). The learning process in biofeedback: Is it feed-forward or feedback? *Biofeedback and Self-Regulation, 11,* 143—156.
Edwards, R.H.T., Melcher, A., Hesser, C.M., Wigertz, O., & Ekelund, L.G. (1972). Physiological correlates of perceived exertion in continous and intermittent exercise with the same average power output. *European Journal of Clinical Investigation, 2,* 108—114.
Fordyce, W. (1976). *Behavioral methods for chronic pain and illness.* St. Louis: Mosby.
Friedlund, A.J., Cottam, G.L., & Fowler, S.C. (1982). In search of the general tension factor: Tensional patterning during auditory stimulation. *Psychophysiology, 19,* 136—145.
Friedlund, A.J., Fowler, S.C., & Pritchard, A. (1980). Striate muscle tensional patterning in frontalis EMG biofeedback. *Psychophysiology, 17,* 47—55.
Funke, N. (1989). Effekte einer therapeutischen Modifikation subjektiver Krankheitsursachen und Kontrollannahmen am Beispiel Migräne. In C. Bischoff & H. Zenz (Eds.), *Patientenkonzepte von Körper und Krankheit.* Bern: Huber.
Gellhorn, E. (1964). Motion and emotion: The role of proprioception in the physiology and pathology of the emotions. *Psychological Review, 71,* 457—472.
Gerber, W.D., Miltner, W., Birbaumer, N., & Lutzenberger, W. (1983). Cephalic vasomotor feedback therapy: A controlled study of migraineurs and normals. In K. Holroyd, B. Schlote, & H. Zenz (Eds.), *Perspectives in research on headache* (pp. 163—170). Toronto/Lewiston, NY: C.J. Hogrefe.
Holroyd, K.A., & Penzien, D.B. (1985). Client variables and the behavioral treatment of recurrent tension headache: A meta-analytic review. *Journal of Behavioral Medicine, 9,* 515—536.
Holroyd, K.A., Penzien, D.B., Hursey, K.G., Tobin, D.L., Rogers, L., Holm, J.E., Marcille, P.J., Hall, J.R., & Chila, A.G. (1984). Change mechanisms in EMG biofeedback training: Cognitive changes underlying improvements in tension headache. *Journal of Consulting and Clinical Psychology, 52,* 1039—1053.
Hudzinski, L.G. (1983). Neck musculature and EMG biofeedback in treatment of muscle contraction headache. *Headache, 23,* 86—90.

Hudzinski, L.G. (1984). The significance of muscle discrimination training in the treatment of chronic muscle contraction headache. *Headache, 24,* 203—210.

Izard, C.E. (1977). *Human emotions.* New York: Plenum Press.

Jacob, R.G., Tuerner, S.N., Szekeley, B.C., & Eidelmann, B.H. (1983). Predicting outcome of relaxation therapy in headaches: The role of "depression." *Behavior Therapie, 14,* 457—465.

Jäger, R., Lischer, S., Münster, B., & Ritz, B. (1976). *Biographisches Inventar zur Diagnose von Verhaltensstörungen (BIV).* Göttingen: Hogrefe.

Kotses, H., & Weiner, H. (1982). Effects of home practice exercises on EMG activity subsequent to biofeedback training. *American Journal of Clinical Biofeedback, 5,* 103—109.

Krampen, G. (1981). *IPC-Fragebogen zu Kontrollüberzeugungen.* Göttingen: Hogrefe.

Lacroix, J.M. (1986). Mechanismus of biofeedback control. In R.J. Davidson, G.E. Schwartz, & D. Shapiro (Eds.), *Consciousness and self-regulation, Vol. 4* (pp. 137—162). New York: Plenum Press.

Laird, J.D. (1984). The real role of facial response in the experience of emotion: A reply to Tourangeau and Ellsworth, and others. *Journal of Personality and Social Psychology, 47,* 909—917.

LeDoux, R. (1984). Cognition and emotion. In M.S. Gazzaniga (Ed.), *Handbook of cognitive neuroscience.* New York: Plenum Press.

Levin, J.R., Marascuilo, L.A., Hubert, L.J. (1978). N=Nonparametric randomisation tests. In Kratochwill, T.R. (Ed.), *Single subject research* (pp. 167—196). New York: Academic Press.

Libo, L.M., & Arnold, G.E. (1983). Does training to criterion influence improvement? A follow-up study to EMG and thermal biofeedback. *Journal of Behavior Medicine, 6,* 397—404.

Mihevic, P.M. (1981). Sensory cues for perceived exertion: A review. *Medicine and Science in Sports and Exercise, 13,* 150—163.

Reinking, R.H., & Hutchings, D. (1981). Follow-up to: "Tension headaches: What form of therapy is most effective?" *Biofeedback and Self-Regulation, 6,* 57—62.

Robinson, C.A. (1980). Cervical spondylosis and muscle contraction headaches. In D.J. Dalessio (Ed.), *Wolff's headache and other head pain.* New York: Oxford University Press.

Sargent, J.D., Solbach, P., & Coyne, L. (1980). Evaluation of a 5-day non-drug training program for headache at the Menninger Foundation. *Headache, 20,* 32—41.

Schwartz, G.E. (1977). Disregulation and systems theory: A biobehavioral framework for biofeedback and behavioral medicine. In N. Birbaumer & H.D. Kimmel (Eds.), *Biofeedback and self-regulation* (pp. 19—48). New York: Wiley.

Stoyva, J., & Budzynski, T. (1974). Cultivated low arousal—An antistress response? In L.V. DiCara (Ed.), *Limbic and autonomic nervous systems research* (pp. 369—394). New York: Plenum.

Tomkins, S.S. (1980). Affect as amplification: Some modifications in theory. In R. Plutchik & H. Kellerman (Ed.), *Emotion. Theory and research and experience, Vol. 1: Theories of emotions* (pp. 141—187). New York: Academic Press.

Traue, H.C., Gottwald, A., Henderson, P.R., & Bakal, D.A. (1985). Nonverbal expressiveness and activity in tension headache sufferers and controls. *Journal of Psychosomatic Research, 29,* 375—381.

Travell, J.G., & Simons, D.G. (1983). *Myofascial pain and dysfunction. The trigger point manual.* Baltimore: Williams & Wilkins.

Ulmer, H.V. (1985). Arbeitsphysiologie—Umweltphysiologie. In R.F. Schmidt & G. Thews (Eds.), *Physiologie des Menschen* (pp. 602—627). Berlin: Springer-Verlag.

Yates, A.J. (1980). *Biofeedback and the modification of behavior.* New York: Plenum Press.

Zipp, P. (1982). Recommendations for the standardization of lead positions in surface electromyography. *European Journal of Applied Physiology, 50*, 41—54.

Author Index

A

AASH Board of Directors 182, 196
ABEL, M. 124, 130, 132
ABRAMOWITZ, S. J. 148, 163, 213, 215
ADAMS, H. E. 191, 198, 200
AD HOC COMMITTEE on Classification of Headache 192, 196
ADLER, C. 181, 197
ADLER, R. 51, 62, 124, 130, 132
AHLES, T. A. 182f., 191, 196f., 204, 214ff.
AHRENS, St. 65, 81, 136, 140, 145, 166ff., 175f.
AKERSON, K. M. 64, 66, 81
ALA-HURULA, V. 190, 196
ALEXANDER, F. 167, 176
ALF, E. 21, 27
ALLAIRE, D. 192, 198
AMERICAN PSYCHIATRIC ASSOCIATION 182, 196
AMSEL, R. 130, 132
ANDERSON, J. A. D. 57, 62, 74, 82
ANDERSON, C. D. 32, 34, 60f.
ANDERSON, L. P. 67, 81
ANDRASIK, F. 14, 27, 148, 161f., 164, 181f., 184ff., 191ff., 195ff., 202, 204, 213f., 215f.
ANWAR, R. 49, 61
APPELBAUM, K. A. 14, 27, 186f., 195, 197, 214f.
ARENA, J. G. 148, 163, 183, 197, 214, 216
ARGELANDER, H. 103ff., 106
ARNOLD, G. E. 204, 217
ARRAYO, P. 74, 81
ATKINSON, J. H. 130ff.
ATTANASIO, V. 194ff.
AWAD, E. A. 74, 81

B

BAER, D. M. 185, 195, 200
BAGG, R. J. 73, 81
BAILEY, S. E. 136, 146
BAKAL, D. A. 25, 34, 45, 47, 49ff., 59f., 61, 87, 106, 148, 164, 191, 196, 203, 214f., 217
BAIR, D. M. 200
BAKER, A. 195, 200
BALL, G. S. 14f., 28
BARBOSA, A. 188, 199
BARD, D. 75, 82
BARLOW, D. H. 187, 196
BARRON, K. G. 187, 195, 197
BASHINSKY, H. S. 21, 27
BASKIN, S. 190f., 199f.
BASMAJIAN, J. V. 4, 10, 12, 75f., 83, 202, 215
BANTZ, M. 149, 163
BECK, A. T. 168, 176
BECKER, M. 187, 200
BECKMANN, D. 140, 145
BELAR, C. D. 78, 81, 203, 215
BELL, N. W. 148, 163, 213, 215
BERNAL, G. A. A. 67, 82, 137, 145
BEYMER, F. 148, 163
BILLE, B. 192ff., 196
BIRBAUMER, N. 10, 12f., 27, 64, 68, 82f., 138, 145, 168, 177, 213, 216
BISCHOFF, C. 13, 15f., 21f., 25f., 27f., 33f., 43, 46ff., 57f., 60f., 68ff., 81, 92, 106, 162f, 191, 195f., 201, 203f., 215
BLACK, A. R. 78, 82
BLAKE, D. D. 193, 196
BLANCHARD, E.B. 14f., 27, 148, 163, 182ff., 191, 195ff., 201, 213ff.
BLASZCYNSKI, A. P. 149, 163
BLOCK, A. 67, 81
BLOVIN, D. 195, 200
BLAME, H. 136, 146
BLUMER, D. 66, 81, 166, 176
BOIS, R. 192, 198
BONICA, J. J. 4, 11
BOTWIN, D. 187, 200
BOWDLER, I. 147
BOXAN, K. 186, 198
BOXTEL, A. van 60f.
BRADY, J. V. 30, 43
BRÄHLER, E. 51, 61, 150, 163
BRADLEY, L. A. 130f.
BRANTLEY, P. J. 191, 200
BROOKS, G. R. 32, 43
BROWN, K. G. 163
BROWN, M. B. 23, 27, 52, 61, 64, 82
BRUHN, P. 188, 197
BUCHSBAUM, M. S. 59, 61
BUCK, R. 30f., 41, 44
BUDZYNSKI, T. 181, 197, 212, 217
BUNNEY, W. E. 59, 61
BURGESS, M. 31, 44
BURKART, S. L. 3, 12
BURKE, E. J. 195ff.
BUSH, C. 11f., 73, 83
BYRNE, D. 30, 44
BYRNE, M. 123, 130ff.

C

CAHN, T. S. 10f., 195, 199
CALLIET, R. 3f., 11f.
CALSYN, D. A. 78, 82
CANNON, W. B. 72, 76, 81
CAPPO, B. M. 209, 216
CARDONA, A. 204, 216
CARMICHAEL, S. W. 3, 12
CARROBLES, J. A. 204, 216
CHAPMAN, S. L. 212, 216
CHELIONT, F. 57, 61
CHEN, A. C. N. 124, 131
CHILA, A. G. 192, 198, 202, 216
CHOROBA, B. 149, 163
CINCIRIPINI, P. M. 14, 27, 71, 82

CLAGHORN, J. L. 192, 199
CLARE, M. H. 9, 12, 76, 83
CLAUS, G. 53f., 61
CLEARY, P.J. 26, 28
CLEMENTS, J. H. 149, 164
COBB, C. R. 73f., 81
COBB, S. 38, 43
COHEN, J. L. 78, 81
COHEN, M. J. 73, 81
COHEN, R. 195, 200
COLEBATCH, J.G. 20, 28
COLLINS, G. A. 73ff., 80f.
COTE, A. 195, 197
COTE, G. 195, 197
COTTAM, G. L. 203, 216
COX, D. 213f., 216
COYNE, L. 187, 200, 204, 217
CRAIG, K. D. 130f.
CRAM, J. R. 3, 5ff., 10ff., 74ff., 81, 191f., 197, 204, 216
CROCKETT, D. J. 130f.
CRONBACH, L. 91, 106

D

DALESSIO, D. J. 188, 200
DAVIDSON, R. J. 10, 12
DAVIS, G. C. 59, 61
DAWSON, E. 123, 132, 136, 146
DAY, C. 47, 62
DEMJEN, S. 191, 196, 214f.
DEPAUW, M. A. 75, 82
DESMEDT, J. E. 20, 27
DHOPESCH, V. P. 49, 61
DIAGNOSTIC AND THERAPEUTIC TECHNOLOGY ASSESSMENT 192, 197
DIAMOND, S. 186f., 193, 197
DIXON, W. J. 23, 27, 52, 61
DOBBINS, K. 192, 199
DOLCE, J. J. 10ff.
DORFMAN, D. D. 21, 27
DOXEY, N. C. 137, 145
DROLET, M. 192, 198
DUBNER, R. 130f.
DUBUISSON, D. 130f.
DUIVENVOORDEN, H. J. 136, 146
DUNN, T. G. 209, 216

DZIOBA, R. B. 137, 145

E

EBNER, H. 53f., 61
EDWARDS, R. H. T. 203, 216
EIDELMAN, B. H. 187, 198, 200, 214, 217
EKELUND, L. G. 203, 216
ELLAM, S. 57, 62
ELLIOT, F. A. 74, 81
ELMAN, N. 187, 200
ENGEL, B. T. 30, 43
ENGELMAN, L. 23, 27, 52, 61
ENGSTROM, D. 6f., 10, 12
EPSTEIN, L. H. 14, 27, 71, 82
EVANS, D. D. 186f., 195, 197
EWERHARD, F. H. 9, 12, 76, 83
EYSENCK 148

F

FAHRENBERG, J. 171, 176
FERENCZI, S. 10, 12
FERGUSON, S. 33, 44
FIGUEROA, J. L. 195, 197
FINLEY, K. H. 46, 61
FIRESTONE, P. 194, 199
FISHER-WILLIAMS, M. 79, 83
FISHMAN, M. 192, 199
FLECK, H. C. 65, 82, 138, 145
FLOR, H. 10, 12, 34, 43, 67, 76, 77f., 82, 138, 145, 149, 163, 167, 175ff.
FLORIN, I. 32, 43f., 186, 198f.
FLOYD, J. W. 59, 61
FOLKINS, C. H. 148, 163, 213, 215
FORD, M. R. 184, 197
FORDYCE, W. E. 17, 27, 67, 82, 138, 144f., 202, 216
FORREST, A. J. 166, 176
FOWLER, R. S. 13ff., 27
FOWLER, S. C. 203, 216
FOX, N. A. 10, 12
FRANE, J. W. 23, 27, 52, 61
FRANKLIN, M. 193, 197
FRANKS, R. D. 60f.
FRANZ, C. 149f., 161, 163
FREEDMAN, R. R. 185, 199
FREEMAN, C. W. 78, 82

FREUDENBERG, G. 32, 43
FRIEDLUND, A. J. 203, 216
FRIEDMAN, A. P. 46, 61, 87, 106, 148, 163
FRÖSCHEN, W. 164
FROMM, G. 130, 132
FRYMOYEN, J. W. 149, 164
FUNKE, N. 213, 216

G

GAINER, J. C. 193, 198
GALEAZZI, R. L. 124, 130, 132
GAMBARO, A. 31, 44
GANDEVIA, S. 20, 28
GARRON, D. C. 131f.
GAUTHIER, J. 192, 195, 197f.
GAYLOR, M. 67, 83
GEISINGER, K. F. 123, 130ff.
GEISSLER, P. 147, 164
GELLHORN, E. 203, 216
GENEST, M. 137, 146
GENTRY, W. D. 67, 82, 130f., 137, 145
GEORG, A. 64, 82
GERBER, W. D. 64, 83, 87, 106, 213, 216
GERHARDS, F. 186, 198
GIBSON, J. G. 80, 83
GIL, K. M. 138, 144f.
GILLIG, S. E. 209, 216
GLASGOW, R. E. 195, 198
GLANZMANN, P. 172, 177
GLAROS, A. G. 73, 82
GLENN, W. V. 64, 82
GLESER, G. C. 91, 106
GLYNN, C. J. 59, 61
GNADE, C. 186, 198
GOLDEN, C. 136, 146
GOLDSTEIN, B. 9, 12
GOUDSWAARD, P. 60f.
GOODELL, H. 47, 62
GOODMAN, J. T. 194, 199
GOTTWALD, A. 25, 34, 45, 148, 164, 203, 217
GRABEL, J. A. 77, 82
GRACELY, R. H. 130f.
GRAHAM, J. R. 46, 61
GRAY, J. A. 41, 44
GREEN, E.E. 181, 199
GRIFFIN, P. 47, 61

Author Index

GROSS, A. 144, 146
GRUSKA, M. 131
GUARNIERI, P. 184, 197
GUILFORD, J. P. 91, 106

H

HAAG, G. 77, 82, 87, 106
HAAS, J. P. 147, 164
HABER, J. D. 191, 198
HABER, L. D. 64, 82
HACK, S. 192, 199
HAESLER, L. 104, 106
HALAR, E. M. 78, 82
HALL, J. R. 192, 198, 202, 216
HAMPEL, R. 171, 176
HANVIK, L. J. 65, 82, 149, 164, 168, 175f.
HARDING, R. H. 74, 82
HARPER, R. G. 60f.
HARRISON, A. 124, 131
HARVEY, L. O. 21, 27
HASENBRING, M. 135ff., 140, 145, 166, 175ff., 187
HAYES, S. C. 187, 196
HAYNES, S. N. 47, 61, 191, 198
HEILBRONN, M. 66, 81, 166, 176
HELLE, P. 169ff., 177
HELM-HYLKEMA, H. 26, 28
HENDERSON, P. R. 25, 34, 45, 148, 164, 203, 217
HERRING, C. L. 49, 61
HESSER, C. M. 203, 216
HILDEBRANDT, G. 59, 62
HILDEBRANDT, J. 149, 163
HILL, M. A. 23, 27, 52, 61
HOBBS, W. R. 213f., 216
HOKANSON, J. E. 31, 44
HOKKANEN, E. 190, 196
HOLE, G. 166
HOLLAENDER, J. 32, 43f.
HOLLINGHEAD, W. H. 3f., 12
HOLM, J. E. 192, 198, 202, 216
HOLMES, D. S. 209, 216
HOLMES, TH. H. 77, 82
HOLROYD, K. A. 148, 164, 182ff., 192, 195f., 198, 200ff., 208, 213ff.
HOOVER, C. W. 38, 44
HOPSON, L. 123, 132

HOPPE, F. 140, 145
HORAL, J. 64, 82
HOWARTH, E. 49, 61
HOYT, W. H. 75f., 83
HUBERT, L. J. 208, 217
HUDZINSKI, L. G. 203f., 216f.
HUI, Y. L. 124, 131
HUNT, H. H. 75, 82
HUNTEN, M. 60, 62, 131
HUNTER, J. W. 20, 27
HUMPHREYS, P. J. 194, 199
HURSEY, K. G. 192, 198, 202, 216
HUSKISSON, E. G. 125, 131
HUTCHINGS, D. 204, 217
HUTCHINSON, G. L. 148, 163, 213, 215

I

IZARD, C. E. 203, 217

J

JACOB, R. G. 187, 198, 214, 217
JACOBSON, E. 17, 26f., 58
JÄGER, R. 39, 44, 213, 217
JARRELL, P. 195, 200
JAY, G. W. 188, 198
JAYASINGHE, W. J. 74, 82
JEANS, M. E. 131f.
JENNRICH, R. I. 23, 27, 52, 61
JOHNSON, E. W. 73, 82
JONES, H. E. 30, 44
JONES, J. M. 190, 199
JONES, L. A. 20, 27
JURISH, S. E. 14, 27, 183, 187, 191, 195, 197, 214, 216

K

KABELA, E. 193, 196
KAGANOV, F. A. 47, 61, 191, 196, 214f.
KAMMER, D. 140, 145
KATZ, F. 33, 44, 131f.
KEEFE, F. J. 78, 82, 137f., 144, 146
KEENE, D. 194, 199
KELLGREN, J. H. 4, 12, 37
KELSEY, J. L. 135, 145
KEMPER, E. 67, 83

KETOVUORI, H. 124, 132
KIELHOLZ, R. 66, 82
KIESLER, D. J. 186, 198
KING, A. 191, 196, 204, 215
KISS, J. 124, 130, 132
KEWMAN, D. 192, 198
KNAPP, T. W. 147, 150, 164, 186, 198f.
KÖHLER, D. M. 152, 165
KÖHLER, TH. 149, 164
KOHLENBERG, R. J. 195, 199
KOTSES, H. 204, 217
KRAFT, G. H. 13ff., 27, 73f., 79, 82f.
KRAMPEN, G. 213, 217
KRAUS, H. 3f., 12
KRAUS, J. 149, 164
KRAUS, W. 41, 44
KRAVITZ, E. 73f., 82
KREMER, E. F. 130ff.
KRÖBER, H. L. 168, 176
KUCZMIERCZYK, A. R. 191, 198
KÜTEMEYER, M. 138, 146, 167, 175, 177
KUDROW, L. 148, 161, 164, 190, 199
KUHL, J. 169ff., 175ff.
KUNKLE, F. C. 46, 61
KUNZEL, M. 188, 200
KUPERMANN, S. 136, 146
KUTNER, M. 4, 12, 76f., 83

L

LABAN, M. M. 73, 82
LABHARDT, A. 65, 82
LACROIX, J. M. 209, 217
LAHUERTA, J. 124, 132
LAIRD, J. D. 26, 27, 203, 217
LAMB, A. M. 78, 83
LANCOURT, J. E. 64, 82
LARGE, R. G. 66, 83, 78
LARGEN, J. W. 192, 199
LARBIG, W. 147, 164
LARSSON, B. 195, 199
LAUNIER, R. 141, 146
LAURIG, W. 20, 28
LAUX, L. 172, 177
LAWLIS, G. F. 149, 164
LAZARUS, R. S. 30, 44, 137, 141, 146

Author Index

LEAVITT, F. 131f., 136, 146
LEDOUX, R. 203, 217
LEFEBVRE, R. C. 213f., 216
LEVI, L. 67, 83
LEVIN, J. R. 208, 217
LEVITON, A. 194, 199
LIBO, L. M. 204, 217
LILLE, F. 57, 61
LIPOWSKI, Z. J. 31, 45
LIPPOLD, O. C. J. 20, 28, 50, 62
LISCHER, S. 39, 44, 213, 217
LOPEZ-IBOR, J. J. 66, 83
LOVE, A. W. 149, 164
LUEKENS, C. A. 73, 81
LUTZENBERGER, W. 213, 216
LYNN, S. J. 185, 199

M

MAHONEY, A. M. 15, 25, 28
MAIANI, G. 124, 132
MANOK, G. 87, 107, 208
MARASCUILO, L. A. 208, 217
MARCHISELLO, P. J. 123, 130ff.
MARCILLE, P. J. 192, 198, 202, 216
MARIENFELD, G. 140, 145
MARKUS, H. 26, 28
MARSCHALL, P. 49, 62, 147
MARTIN, J. E. 191, 196, 204, 215
MARTIN, P. R. 47, 62, 182, 190, 199
MARTINEZ-LAGE, J. M. 124, 132
MARUFA, T. 166, 177
MATARAZZO, J. D. 91, 106
MATAS, M. 166, 177
MATHEW, N. T. 188f., 191, 199
MATHEW, R. J. 192, 199
MATHEWS, A. M. 47, 62
MATUS, J. 14f., 28
MAYER, C. 166
McCARRAN, M. S. 193, 196
McCLOSKEY, D. I. 20, 28
McCREARY, L. 123, 132, 136, 146

McCOY, C. E. 149, 164
McGILL, J. C. 123, 149, 164
McGRATH, P. J. 130f., 194, 199
McGUIGAN, F. J. 26, 28
McMASTER, G. W. 57, 62
McNICOL, D. 21f., 28
MEAD, T. 188, 198
MECHANIC, D. 162, 164
MEICHENBAUM, D. H. 137, 146, 168, 177
MEISSNER, S. J. 31, 44
MELCHER, A. 203, 216
MELGAARD, B. 188, 197
MELIN, L. 195, 199
MELZACK, R. 123ff., 130ff., 136, 146
MENDL, G. 123f., 132
MENSE, S. 25, 28
MERSKEY, H. 65, 83
MIDAX, D. 123, 132
MIHEVIC, P. M. 203, 217
MILTNER, W. 64, 83, 213, 216
MINUCHIN, S. 66, 83
MONGUILLOT, J. 195, 200
MONTROSE, D. 186f., 197
MOONEY, D. 47, 61
MOONEY, V. 149, 164
MOORE, M. E. 73, 82
MORAN, C. C. 26, 28
MOREIRA, A. 188, 199
MÜLLER, H. 124, 130, 132
MÜLLER, K.-J. 16, 195, 201
MÜNSTER, B. 39, 44, 213, 217
MULLANEY, D. J. 181, 197
MULLINIX, V. J. 192, 199
MURPHY, R. W. 66, 83
MURRAY, J. B. 149, 161, 164
MYLLYLA, V. 190, 196

N

NALIBO B. D. 73, 81
NEFF, D. F. 184ff., 191, 196f., 204, 213ff.
NELSON, K. 21, 27
NELSON, R. O. 187, 196
NICASSIO, D. M. 163
NIGL, A. J. 79, 83
NOBLE, J. 195, 198
NOEWEN, A. 11f.
NORTON, B. 192, 199

NOUWEN, A. 72ff., 83
NUNES, S. 188, 199

O

OHNHAUS, E. E. 51, 62
O'KEEFE, D. 182, 191, 197
OLESEN, J. 188, 197
OOSTDAM, E. M. M. 136, 146
ORLEBEKE, J. F. 26, 28
ORTON, K. 191, 200
OSMON, D. 136, 146
OSTFELD, 46, 61

P

PADRAZA, E. 66, 81
PAGE, S. 57, 62
PAIGE, A. B. 78, 82
PAIVA, T. 188, 199
PALLMEYER, T. P. 183, 197, 214, 216
PARISE, M. 47, 61
PASSIAS, J. N. 75, 82
PASSCHIER, J. H. 26, 28
PAUL, R. 149, 163
PECK, C. L. 79, 83, 149, 164
PENNEBAKER, J. W. 38, 44, 94, 106, 150, 164
PENZIEN, D. B. 182f., 186, 192, 198, 201f., 213f., 216
PEREZ, F. 191, 199
PETER, K. 124, 132
PETERS, U. H. 147, 164
PETRIK, M. 186, 198
PHILIPS, C. 46f., 60, 62, 87, 106, 148, 164, 190, 199
PIKOFF, H. 16, 28
POBBINS, D. H. 75, 82
PÖLLMANN, L. 59, 62
PÖLDINGER, W. 167, 177
PÖNTINEN, P. J. 124, 132
PÖPPEL, E. 124, 132
PONSOR, S. E. 209, 216
POPE, G. 66, 81
POTTER, E. K. 20, 28
POZNIAK-PATEWICZ, E. 60, 62
PRATT, M. 195, 200
PRICE, J. P. 4, 9, 11f., 75f., 83
PRIETO, E. J. 123, 130ff.
PRITCHARD, A. 203, 216
PROCACCI, P. 59, 62

PROKOP, CK. 130f.
PRKACHIN, K. M. 130f.

R

RAAB, W. 3f., 12
RABIN, S. 31, 44
RABKIN, R. VII, VIII
RACZYNSKI, J. M 10ff.
RADICHAK, L. D. 148, 163
RAPOPORT, A. 190f., 199f.
RADVILA, A. 124, 130, 132
READING, A. E. 130ff.
REHM, L. P. 67, 81
REICH, W. 167, 177
REINKING, R. H. 204, 217
RENELLI, D. 188, 198
REUVENI, U. 191, 199
REYNOLDS, R. 195, 200
RHODES, M. L. 64, 82
RICHARDSON, F. C. 33, 43
RICHTER, H. E. 140, 145
RICHTER, I. L. 194, 199
RIETH, F. 147
RINZLER, S. 4, 9, 12
RITZ, B. 39, 44, 213, 217
ROBERTS, A. H. 192, 198
ROBINSON, C. A. 26, 28, 204, 217
ROCCHIO, P. D. 136, 146
RODBARD, S. 4, 12
RODICHOK, L. D. 183ff., 195ff., 204, 213ff.
ROGERS, L. 192, 198, 202, 216
ROJAHN,M J. 186, 198
ROSEN, G. M. 195, 198
ROSEN, J. C. 149, 164
ROSENSTIEL, A. K. 137, 144, 146
ROSKIES, E. 137, 146
ROY, R. 166, 177
RUDY, TH. E. 149, 165
RUGH, J. D. 49, 62
RUESCH, S. 31, 44
RUNYON, D. G. 75, 82
RUSSE, T. C. 4, 12, 76f., 83

S

SAINSBURY, P. 80, 83
SANAVIO, E. 124, 132
SANDERS, S. H. 138, 146

SANTACREU, J. 204, 216
SAPER, J. R. 190f., 199
SARGENT, J. D. 181, 187, 199f., 204, 217
SAUERMANN, G. 13, 15, 20, 26ff., 49, 60, 203
SAUNDERS, N. L. 183, 197, 214, 216
SCHANDLER, S. L. 73, 81
SCHAFFNER, P. 172, 177
SCHEER, J. W. 150, 163
SCHEMM, R. 187, 200
SCHLOTE, B. M. VII, 15, 26, 34, 44, 46ff., 50ff., 62, 191, 199, 207f., 212
SCHMIDT, R. F. 20, 25, 28
SCHULTZ, U. 138, 146, 167, 175, 177
SCHWARTZ, G. E. 34, 44, 215, 217
SEITZ, P. F. D. 32, 44
SELBY, D. 149, 164
SELG, H. 171, 176
SEMRAD, S. E. 75, 82
SESSLE, B. J. 131
SHAFFER, F. 75, 82
SHEFTELL, F. 190f., 199f.
SIFNEOS, P. E. 30, 44
SILLANPAA, M. 192, 200
SIMONS, D. J. 47, 60, 62
SIMONS, D. G. 203, 209, 217
SMITH, B. A. 124, 132
SOLA, A. E. 4, 12
SOLBACH, P. 187, 200, 204, 217
SOLBERG, W. K. 49, 62
SOLINGER, J. W. 77, 83,
SONTOS, J. 188, 199
SOVAK, N. 188, 200
SPENSLEY, J. 148, 163, 213, 215
SPIELBERGER, C. D. 172, 177
STEGER, J. C. 5, 12, 60f., 74ff., 81
STEIN, C. 123f., 132
STERNBACH, R. A. 31, 45, 66, 83, 161, 164, 188, 200
STEVENS, S. S. 14, 28
STILSON, D. W. 14f., 28
STOKES, T. F. 185, 195, 200

STOKVIS, B. 31, 45
STOYVA, J. 181, 197, 212, 217
STRAUB, R. 166
STROEBEL, C. F. 184, 197
STRONG, P. 184, 197
STUPPARD, R. 64, 82
SURWIT, R. S. 78, 82
SUTKUS, B. J. 148, 161, 164
SWANSON, D. W. 166, 177
SWANSON, W. M. 166, 177
SWEETMAN, B. J. 57, 62, 74, 82
SZAREK, B. L. 184, 197
SZEKELY, B. C. 187, 198, 200, 214, 217

T

TEDERS, S. J. 148, 163, 182f., 187, 195, 197, 214, 216
TEEVAN, R. C. 148, 163
TEIZEIRA, J. 188, 199
TELNER, P. 33, 44
TERRENCE, C. 130, 132
TEUFEL, R. 64, 138
THOMAS, D. 213, 216
THOMAS, M. 166, 177
TOBIN, D. L. 192, 195, 198, 200, 202, 216
TOBOREK, J. B. 23, 27
TOMKINS, S. S. 203, 217
TOPOREK, J. D. 52, 61
TORGENSON, W. S. 123ff., 130, 132, 136, 146
TRAUE, H. C. 15f., 25ff., 33f., 41, 43, 45ff., 57ff., 61f, 64, 68ff., 81, 92, 106, 138, 148, 164, 191, 196, 203f., 215, 217
TRAVELL, J. G. 4, 9, 12, 203, 209, 217
TREEDE, R. D. 131
TROY, A. 130f.
TUERNER, S. N. 214, 217
TUNIS, M. M. 29, 45, 47, 63
TURK, D. C. 10, 12, 34, 43, 68, 77, 82, 137, 146, 149, 163, 165, 167f., 177
TURKAT, I. D. 191, 200
TURNER, J. 123, 132, 136, 146
TURNER, S. M. 187, 198

U
ULMER, H. V. 26, 28, 204, 217
URBAN, R. T. 73, 81

V
VAN DER HEIDE, L. H. 130f.
VANSELOV, B. 149, 164
VARRUSKA, G. W. 33, 44
VORKAUF, H. 124, 130, 132
VRIES, H. A. de 73f., 81

W
WALL, P. D. 136, 146
WALTERS, E. D. 181, 199
WARING, E. M. 136, 146
WATT, K. C. 75, 82
WEATHERHEAD, A. D. 148, 165
WEEKS, R. 190f., 199f.
WEIL, N. 209, 216
WEINER, H. 29, 45, 204, 217
WEISZ, G. M. 136, 146
WERDER, D. S. 187, 200
WESTBROOK, T. 186, 198
WHITE, B. 138, 146
WIGERTZ, O. 203, 216
WILLIAMS, R. B. 78, 82
WILLIAMS, R. L. 4, 12
WILLIAMSON, D. 195, 200
WILTSE, L. L. 136, 146
WINER, B. J. 95, 106
WITTKOWER, E. D. 31f., 44f.
WÖRZ, R. 190, 200
WOLF, R. S. 66, 83
WOLF, S. 4, 10, 12
WOLF, S. L. 75f., 83
WOLF-CRAMER, B. 16, 28, 30, 63
WOLFF, H. G. 29, 45ff., 60f., 63, 65, 77, 82, 147
WOLKIND, S. N. 166, 176

Y
YATES, A. J. 212, 217

Z
ZAJONC, R.B. 26
ZENZ, H. 34, 43, 49, 57, 61f., 87, 92, 107, 162ff., 208
ZERSSEN, D. V. 140, 146, 152, 165
ZIPP, P. 20, 28, 50, 63, 209, 218
ZOIKE, E. 64, 82
ZUCKERMANN, M. 92, 106
ZUNG, W. K. 172, 177

Subject Index

achievement motivation 26
action-control 170
affect 32
− see emotion
affective communication test 42
alexithymia 30, 41, 103
− see internalization
− see inhibition
atypical facial pain 130
autonomic feedback training 182f.

back pain 131
− low back pain 33, 64ff., 135ff., 149, 166ff.
− see myogenic back pain
− operant model 67
− predictors 135
behavioral analysis 87ff.
behavioral suppression 30ff.
− see inhibition
biofeedback
− age and 186
− alternative delivery modes 194f., 204ff.
− autogenic feedback training 182
− cybernetics 214
− see EMG-biofeedback
− see headache
− internal 214
− maintenance of treatment effects 184f.
− meta-analyses 182f.
− non-contingent 183
− optical 17
− pediatric application 193f.
− physiological vs. psychological learning 191, 201ff.
− psychological variables 80, 187, 213
− self-regulation in 214
− thermal 182
− treatment efficacy 182
− treatment mechanisms 80, 190f., 201ff.
− vasomotor 182
bruxism 33

children 43, 192
cluster headache 197
cognitive therapy 185f.

conversion 65, 136, 149
coping 30, 37, 68, 72, 92, 163
countertransference 99

daily hassles 38
depression 66, 136ff., 148ff., 166ff., 187, 213
− see headache
diathesis-stress model 67, 168
− see stress

EMG-assessment 6ff.
− field registration 34ff., 46ff., 52, 208
− resting level 73
EMG-biofeedback
− generalization of effects 204ff.
− indication 202ff.
− myogenic headache 203ff.
− portable 203, 205ff.
− proprioception 42, 203ff.
− self-efficacy 202
− self-regulation 94, 214
− thresholds 206ff.
− voluntary control of muscle tension 42, 203
emotion 3f., 25, 30ff., 96, 137, 203f.
− anger 31
− see depression
− see expressive behavior
− guilt 31
− skill training 33, 42
exertion, physical and mental 25
expressive behavior 29, 34ff., 96
− smiling 39
− facial signs 32

family system 66, 161
− see parental upbringing

gate-control theory 136

headache
− biofeedback 178ff.
− biofeedback vs. medical treatment 189
− cluster 187
− cognitive therapy 185f.

- depression 187, 213
- diagnosis 42, 87ff., 118ff.
- epidemiology 64, 135
- etiology 29ff., 68, 93
- medical treatment 188f.
- medication rebound headache 190
- menstrual 187
- see migraine
- see muscle contraction headache
- see myogenic headache
- pediatric 43, 192f.
- prevention 43
- psychophysiology 64ff., 138
- relaxation therapy 182ff.
- see tension headache

headache assessment
- diary 208
- interview 91ff., 107, 208
- seee pain measurement
- questionnaire 208

inhibition 29, 37, 41
internalization 30
- see emotion
- see inhibition

life events 38
low back pain 64ff., 80
- see back pain
maladaption 29
McGill Pain Questionnaire 123ff.
- German version 123ff.
medical treatment 188f.
medication rebound headache 190
menstrual headache 187
migraine 147, 194
- autonomic feedback training 182f.
- thermal biofeedback 182f.
- vasomotor biofeedback 182f.
muscle activity/tension
- classical conditioning 25, 34, 43, 67
- see conditioning
- dysfunctional 29, 48, 68ff.
- EMG-assessment 4, 39
- see EMG-biofeedback
- EMG field registration 46ff., 208
- EMG-scanning 5ff.
- emotion 3f., 25, 29ff.
- see emotion
- frontalis 6f., 15

- gravitational influences 3, 4, 9
- headache 25, 29ff., 39, 201ff.
- ischemia 4, 25
- movement 25
- neuromuscular patterns 3ff., 9ff., 29ff., 68ff.
- operant conditioning 25, 34, 43, 67
- paraspinalis 6ff.
- perception 13ff.
- posture 3ff., 9ff., 25
- site 3ff., 9ff., 29ff.
- static vs. dynamic 204, 212
- symmetry 3ff., 9ff.
- trapezius 6ff., 15
- voluntary control 21, 203
muscle contraction headache 203ff.
- EMG-biofeedback 203ff.
- see myogenic headache
myofascial pain syndrom 33
myogenic back pain
- biomechanical model 3, 4, 9
- diathesis stress model 4, 64ff.
- gravitational influences 3
- see low back pain
- mechanical sources 4
- neuromuscular patterns 3ff., 9ff., 64ff.
- physical therapy 4
- posture 3ff., 9ff.
myogenic headache 191, 203ff.
- achievement motivation 26
- diagnosis 190f., 212
- EMG-biofeedback 201ff.
- frontalis muscle activity 15
- see muscle contraction headache
- proprioception 13ff.
- signal detection analysis of muscle activity 13ff.
- static overload 204
- see tension headache
- trapezius muscle activity 15
- trigger points 48
myogenic pain 29, 33, 47, 64
- irritation of muscle tissue 4
- ischemia 4, 25, 48, 203f.
- see myogenic back pain
- see myogenic headache
- referred pain 9, 203

neonates 43
- see children

Subject Index

pain
- chronic 135ff., 147ff.
- classification 65
- cognitive dimension 123f., 137, 169
- descriptors 126ff.
- management 88, 178ff.
- motivational dimension 123f.
- nociceptors 48
- proneness 72, 166
- referred 9, 203
- risc factors 41
- sensory dimension 123f.
- treatment 42, 100, 178ff., 182f.
- treatment efficacy 182ff.

pain measurement
- cross-cultural comparison 131
- McGill Pain Questionnaire 123ff.
- multidimensional 123ff.

parental upbringing 39
- see children

pediatric headache 192f.
- see children

personality factors
- denial 159
- see emotion
- hysteria 136, 148ff.
- see inhibition
- motivation 168
- personality 142ff., 166, 187
- repression 30
- risk factors 41
- self-disclosure 42
- self-efficacy 99, 202
- socialization 34
- see social support

physical symptoms 32, 59, 150ff.
physical therapy 4
proprioception
- emotion 25, 203f.
- exertion, physical and mental 25

- frontal muscle activity 13ff.
- functions 203ff.
- levels of information processing 203
- magnitude production method 14f.
- perceived effort 203
- signal detection analysis 13ff.

psychoanalysis 65, 138

recreation 39, 116
rheumatoid arthritis 32

self-regulation 94, 214
sexuality 39, 113
signal detection analysis 13ff.
social activity 150
social environment 30
- see social stress
social support 37
- as protective system 38

stress
- coping with 68
- see diathese-stress model
- disorders 29
- natural 34
- report 46, 51ff.
- social 30ff.

tension headache
- as depression equivalent 202
- behavioral interventions 181ff., 201ff.
- diagnosis 190
- EMG-biofeedback 182ff., 201ff.
- see muscle contraction headache
- see myogenic headache
- operant conditioning 202

thermal biofeedback 182f.
trigeminal neuralgia 130

vasomotor biofeedback 182f.